Our Own Capabilities

Clinlcal nurse managers taking a strategic approach to service improvements

Marion Macalpine
Sheila Marsh

Co-ordinated by
Roma Iskander,
King's Fund Nursing Developments Programme

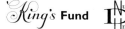

Published by
King's Fund Publishing
11–13 Cavendish Square
London W1M 0AN
Tel: 0171 307 2400

ISBN   1 85717 099 7

A CIP catalogue record for this book is available from the British
Library.

Distributed by: Bournemouth English Book Centre (BEBC)
PO Box 1496
Poole
Dorset BH12 3YD
Tel: 0800 262260
Fax: 0800 262266

Cover photograph: Telegraph Colour Library

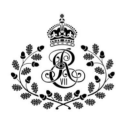

Contents

Foreword

This important publication should be essential reading for all those who are working to introduce improvements at the point of service or education delivery in healthcare. It aims to share the experiences of clinical leaders in nursing development units (NDUs) and to discuss the implications of these experiences for service improvement. The sharing of lessons learned is an essential ingredient in handling change effectively and helping us all to become more reflective practitioners.

We live in a world of continuous change, characterised by repeated cycles of innovation, experimentation, implementation, consolidation and evaluation. We should not be concerned with change for its own sake but as a necessary ingredient in the constant improvement of the service we offer. Of all these stages in the cycle, implementation and consolidation – 'making it happen and making it stick' – are the most difficult. How many really good innovations do we see fall by the wayside when the innovator leaves! Integrating the improved service into the system is the crucial test. There is much in this publication that seeks to address this issue.

The other powerful message is that if clinical leaders adopt an organisational as well as a professional approach to change, and look outwards as well as inwards when planning and implementing change, they have potential to create an environment of continuous improvement.

Peter Griffiths
Director
King's Fund Management College

Acknowledgements

The King's Fund would like to thank the staff of the following NDUs:

Cartmel Ward, Prestwich Hospital, Manchester

Charlton Road Health Centre, Andover

Clare House, St George's Hospital, London

Day Ward, Worthing Hospital, Worthing

Maternity Unit, Royal Bournemouth Hospital, Bournemouth

Ward 22, Newcastle General Hospital, Newcastle upon Tyne

Stepney Neighbourhood Nursing Team, Steels Lane Health Centre, London

Strelley Health Centre, Nottingham

The willingness of the staff on these units to share information, and the time they gave for interviews and discussions, have made this publication possible.

Chapter I
Introducing change for service improvement

This study is based on nurses' experiences and is aimed primarily at nurse managers. It focuses on ways of *managing* nursing practice so that patients and clients have a better experience. The study did not set out to be prescriptive or to act as a training guide. What it aims to do is to collect the experience of nurses, patients or clients, managers and other professionals and to generalise from this experience in order to take and generate the best ideas for nurses to manage service improvements. These are summarised at the end of each chapter and on pages 76-80.

In recent years there has been much attention given to 'managing change' both inside and outside the National Health Service (NHS). This study deliberately focuses on those changes which aim to improve the service offered to users (patients and clients). This chapter introduces the eight NDUs used in the study to examine the experiences of nurses who have been involved in projects aimed specifically at achieving service improvement. Fuller descriptions of these units are given in Appendix 1.

The study focuses on:

- service development at unit or operational team level (rather than trust- or district-led initiatives)
- a managerial rather than a clinical perspective
- introducing and embedding innovations
- crucial related issues such as nurses' roles and self-image, the part played by female/male dynamics and by ethnic diversity.

'Successful' service development refers to a change which:

- improves the experiences of patients and clients
- produces organisational change to support clinical changes
- is sufficiently embedded to become part of on-going practice and so can be sustained over time.

The focus is on changes at the unit or team level because this reflects the origin of the NDUs, but the study also explores the reality of attempting change for individual nurse managers[1] in the cost-conscious, pressured work environment of the NHS.

The case studies

All the case studies are NDUs. They are not necessarily typical of other nursing environments in that, by seeking NDU status, they have chosen to innovate, to generalise best practice and to develop the nursing contribution to service delivery. Nonetheless, their experiences are very mixed and reflect the diversity of the NHS. All the units visited were involved in an array of changes of which only one key example was selected for study.

Individual and group interviews were carried out at different levels in the units, 'slicing' through the hierarchy where possible to include managers, doctors, all nursing grades, and service users. This gave a variety of perspectives on each change. Despite the increasing number of men in nursing jobs and of women in medical positions, in the case studies all the key consultants and doctors were men and all the clinical leaders but one were women. Several male nurses were interviewed, but it was striking how few Black staff were involved in the units, at least on the day shifts when the visits took place.

The study did not start with a theory of change management to explore in practice. Instead, it aimed at drawing on the case studies to present the principles and issues which emerged *directly from the experiences of the people involved* in the changes. The material presented in the following chapters is therefore based on fieldwork, and describes and assesses the service improvement projects and their progress. Each chapter analyses the case information in different ways in order to draw helpful principles and illustrate positive practices. The analysis also highlights some difficulties the units experienced, most of which were identified by the staff themselves, and ways of avoiding these difficulties.

Initial analysis of the case information

The case profiles summarised in Table 1 identify:

- the service improvement
- the specific type of change required to achieve the service improvement
- the 'triggers' for the change
- how the change was introduced.

Case study	Service improvement	Change focus	Triggers	Approach
Mental health	Improved staff morale	Staff development projects	Internal	Project team; systematic
Anorexia	New outpatient service	Variety of nurse-led treatments	Internal	Political; managerial; staff development
Health visiting	Pubic health focus	Community-based projects; work re-organisation	External	Pilot projects; gradual build-up
Neighbourhood healthcare	Proper nourishment of Bangladeshi children	Role of professional knowledge; empowering service users	Internal/external	Activity workshops; joint work with service users
Orthopaedic trauma	Improved continuity of care and acceleration of rehabilitation process	Case management	Internal/external	Staff development; research; documentation
District nursing	Continuity of care for patients moving into hospital	District nurses as primary nurses in a hospital setting	Internal	Staff development; stakeholder involvement; documentation
Day ward	Dedicated services for day treatments and procedures	Nurse-led unit and nurse-administered treatments	Internal/external	Staff development; work planning; computer records
Maternity	New facility for 'low-risk' women	Midwife-led service; service user involvement	External	Stakeholder involvement; overnight move to a new unit; monitoring and audit

Table 1: A summary of the case profiles

The case information is analysed, first, to identify the *type* of service improvement the units were working on, the changes involved and what can be learnt from this. Second, the *triggers* for the changes are examined to assess the extent to which they were initiated from outside the unit or from within it, among the staff. Third, the analysis looks at *how* the changes were managed, whether they were introduced in stages or all in one go, and at what pace.

Type of service improvement

The units studied were very diverse in terms of the work environment, the type of treatment or service offered and the patients or clients being served. However, all the service improvements involved one or more of the following elements:

- new or extended services
- expanding/developing the role of nurses, resulting in greater opportunity for decision-making
- staff development
- changes in beliefs or values underlying the service improvement
- system or process changes affecting the way in which the improvement was effected.

New or extended services were least common in the case studies, whereas an extension of the role of nurses was a feature of most of them. All the units are deeply involved in staff development, by virtue of being NDUs, and in all the case studies this was a key element in initiating changes. In implementing changes, several units were acting upon different beliefs and values from those traditionally held about health and sickness and about patient participation in decisions affecting their treatment. All the units visited were involved in some changes to their organisational system and procedures as part of their service improvement project. Some saw the system changes as the main focus of the service improvement.

The nurses involved in the changes found that whatever aspect of service improvement their work focused on, whether a 'micro' or 'macro' type of change, *the various elements they had to deal with were linked*:

- the extended service improvement required new roles and/or attention to systems
- new processes required a review of roles and structures in the units

4

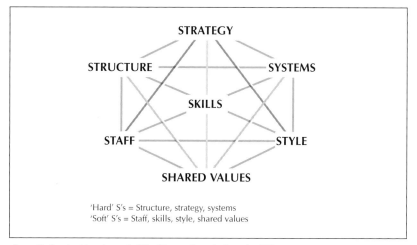

STRATEGY

STRUCTURE ——— SYSTEMS

SKILLS

STAFF ——— STYLE

SHARED VALUES

'Hard' S's = Structure, strategy, systems
'Soft' S's = Staff, skills, style, shared values

Source: R. Pascale, *Managing on the Edge.* Harmondsworth: Penguin, 1990.

Fig. 1: *The 'Seven S' model*

- working to new or refocused values involved procedures as well as skills
- to acquire new knowledge and skills, staff development seemed to be a pre-requisite of change.

This interconnection and the need to forecast and manage its implications were the focus of research conducted at Harvard University on change in organisations, from which the 'Seven S' model[2] was derived (*see* Figure 1). In this model, the term 'systems' refers to the broad interconnections within an organisation, not just the organisational procedures; the term 'style' refers to management style. The model shows the link between the key elements of management, some of which have long been recognised, such as strategy or systems, and others which the researchers identified more recently in Japanese organisations, such as shared values. One conclusion from this research was that successful change requires systematic attention to all these elements.

Interestingly, the Harvard researchers noted that, traditionally, private sector managers focus most on the 'hard' S's and pay insufficient attention to the 'soft' S's. In the public sector there has been criticism that the focus has been the opposite of this. While nurses seem to focus most on systems, shared values, staff and skills, they tend to pay less attention to strategy, structures and style. Table 2 illustrates how the case studies relate to the 'Seven S' model.

Case study	Strategy	Systems	Structures	Staff	Style	Shared values	Skills	Incremental/ radical change	Fast/slow change
Mental health	SF	SF	LF	IF	SF	LF	IF	INCR	S
Anorexia	SF	IF	SF	IF	IF	IF	IF	RAD	F
Health visiting	LF	SF	LF	IF	LF	IF	SF	INCR	S
Neighbourhood healthcare	SF	LF	LF	IF	LF	IF	IF	INCR	S
Orthopaedic trauma	IF	IF	LF	SF	LF	SF	IF	INCR	S
District nursing	LF	IF	LF	IF	LF	SF	SF	INCR	S
Day ward	LF	IF	IF	IF	IF	SF	SF	BOTH	F
Maternity	IF	IF	SF	IF	SF	IF	IF	RAD	F

Table 2: *Service improvement focus and approach in the case studies*

Note: IF = important focus; SF = some focus; LF = little focus

Triggers for change

In identifying what brought about the changes in the units and how much control nurses had in planning and implementing a service improvement project, it was striking that most were self-initiated. The key motivation for the changes was more to do with improving practice and 'professionalism' than with cost reduction or responding to a broader agenda within the NHS, such as meeting the expectations of purchasers. This may not be surprising since NDUs have chosen to be practice innovators and to take a developmental track. There was also, not surprisingly given the emphasis on improving practice, a clear commitment to offering a better service to patients and clients, whether in their relationship with nurses or within the broader context of policy development.

How the changes were introduced

Some changes were introduced gradually by building upon existing practices, sending up 'trial balloons'[3] or trying out new ideas as pilot projects. This approach may be termed 'incremental'. In other cases, changes were introduced as a 'big bang', a more immediate and 'radical' approach.

What seems clear from the case studies is that both approaches to change may be appropriate. Table 2 incorporates a summary of the approaches adopted by the nurse managers in the units studied. Box 1 outlines examples of incremental change. In several cases, incremental change *followed* radical change because of the need to refocus and regroup after major disruption, as in the case of the Maternity Unit changes described in Box 2.

Box 1

In the Health Visitor Unit, a variety of ways of involving the community in identifying the most important health issues were tried out as experiments, using an *incremental* approach by building upon a mixture of activities over time.

In the Mental Health Unit, a series of development projects was set up to foster staff motivation.

> ## Box 2
>
> In the Maternity Unit, the introduction of a midwife-led service involved *radical* changes, including moving to a new building and the midwives taking on major new responsibilities without a break in the service being offered to patients. The clinical leader reported that: 'The initial change was managed quite well; however, because of that timescale we didn't actually manage the carry-through very well, although change was managed, well, it happened, there were aspects of it that were very good. But I think that it was a year down the line that we started to see the fragmentation appearing down the edges where people were a little bit gobsmacked by it all.'
>
> By contrast, the unit is also planning the integration of the hospital and community midwife teams, which involves bringing together teams with different cultures, roles, hours and rewards. The process of integrating the two teams has been planned as an *incremental* process, designed to take five years. 'I don't disagree with abrupt change,' said the clinical leader. 'It was successful once, but with incremental change you have more chance of taking the majority of staff with you.' The first step is for hospital midwives to cover community clinics, and there will be a forum for staff to voice their opinions. It is hoped that this approach will identify and change the stereotyped views that hospital midwives may have of community midwives, and vice versa. On a practical level, it will also enable the participants to deal with the small things that matter to individuals, such as how they claim their mileage.

Over-reliance on an incremental approach to change, however, can make people feel that nothing is really happening and lead to less being achieved than may have been possible by including some radical action. In addition, if changes are implemented too slowly they have a tendency to be overtaken by events and/or to become invisible unless the overall goals and direction are clearly stated and visible throughout. As illustrated by the examples in Box 3, maintaining momentum and keeping people 'on board' are vital in the incremental approach.

Summary

Whether the approach to introducing change is incremental or radical, the case studies show that *from the outset the whole process needs to be visualised within a broad strategic context, with clear goals.* What is required

Box 3

In the Health Visitor Unit, because of rapid and continuous structural changes, uncertainty, the absence of consistent senior management support and the departure of key 'champions' of the changes, there was a risk that the promising new projects would simply become a series of pilot projects which would gradually disappear. Initially, the unit had carried out its pilot projects with no plan for how they were going to be evaluated and embedded if they were successful.

In the Orthopaedic Trauma Unit, the gradual introduction of changes made the phases that were successful less visible to staff. This fostered a sense that little progress was being made and reduced the commitment of staff to the changes. A year was spent doing preparatory work for case management, which included a staff development programme, but there was a feeling that the change process was going on and on. Factors contributing to the delay included hospital reorganisation, problems of planning staff time and slow progress in reaching agreement on the formal research project before implementation. 'We've been waiting a year,' commented one of the nurses. The project ran the risk of running out of steam and losing the support of key managers because it had taken so long. It was also becoming difficult to maintain enthusiasm for the project among those directly involved in it.

In the Day Ward Unit, there was a gradual increase in the type of treatments offered. On a day-to-day basis, there was clear and effective planning by the nurses to ensure that each patient had sufficient time and a relaxed environment, sometimes against the wishes of doctors who wanted to squeeze in last-minute patients. However, there did not appear to be a plan for how the inevitable increase in the numbers of people to be treated was going to be dealt with in the longer term.

is a strategy that takes into account not only the systems but also the staff, the structures and the management style (*see* Figure 1).

Within this overall approach to change, getting the speed of the actual change right for the people involved is crucial to prevent them being overwhelmed with too rapid a change or bored with a process that never seems to end.

What has emerged from the case studies is that the change strategist[4] (in these cases, usually the ward sister or clinical leader) needs to *plan for the change and try to envisage how it will affect the people involved.*

The strategist also needs to communicate fully at all stages with everyone involved, paying particular attention to people still on the edge of the change so that they know what to expect and when. These skills were developed through a learning process over time, through discussions and analysis with colleagues, facilitated by the King's Fund project officers.

The comments made by the clinical leader of the Maternity Unit on strategic planning indicate that the effort required to make changes had not been predicted: 'That's something to be learned: trying to have a more strategic approach as a manager... On reflection, we should have closed the ward... It was very busy, senior midwives had to learn to cope with that responsibility. This provided momentum for the next few months. Staff were very committed, they had evening meetings outside duty hours and stayed late. This lasted 9 to 12 months. Then staff became disgruntled. They were tired and they did not want to change any more. People started floundering.'

Another clinical leader acknowledged the lack of strategic planning: 'Setting up the NDU was seen as a way to recruit staff to a hard-to-recruit area ... [there was] no framework of stages we need to go through ... that [process of] learning has been invaluable for me.'

The initial analysis of the case studies has highlighted the key issues in introducing changes aimed at service improvement:

- successful change requires *systematic attention to all the aspects* of the change and recognition of their interconnectedness; the 'Seven S' model may be useful as a checklist for what needs to considered about aspects of the change being planned
- drawing up an *explicit strategic plan* at the outset helps a great deal, particularly in terms of deciding whether the radical or incremental approach is best and identifying the strengths and weaknesses of each approach
- consideration needs to be given to *the speed of the change and its impact* on all the people involved, especially the recipients of change[5] who are usually the people who will need to carry out the new activities
- communication about the change needs to *spell out the process of the change as well as the content of the change* (i.e., its clinical or practice content).

The case studies also underlined the importance of outside factors in managing change. These will be considered in more depth in Chapter 2.

Chapter 2
Actively managing change

The first chapter discussed the issues that nurse managers need to consider when planning and carrying through changes aimed at service improvement. The demand for more planning and a more strategic approach is a common one, but what does this mean for individual managers at practice level? This issue is examined below by drawing on actual experiences of managing change from the perspectives of staff, managers, patients and clients. It opens with a summary of what appeared to be common to these experiences, including those approaches that seemed to be effective and those that did not. It then explores the effective approaches in more detail.

Common approaches in managing change

The following approaches to managing change appeared to be effective, across very different sites and whatever the type of change involved:

- where the change was clearly conceived and tightly managed as a specific project by a person in a well-defined management role, usually the clinical leader
- where nurse expertise and power were used and clearly demonstrated by the unit in implementing the change
- where the change introduced was in tune with specific external factors
- where communication with users and all relevant staff was a key component of managing the change.

In general, problems in implementing and embedding change arose in one or more of the following situations:

- where there was more than usual uncertainty in the organisational environment, such as in the early stages of trust formation or with an impending merger (managing uncertainty was best tackled where a unit had adopted the effective approaches listed above)
- where the clinical leader was reluctant or ambivalent about playing a specific *management* role

- where the clinical leader viewed specific changes in isolation, rather than seeing them as linked to a continuous process of improvement that involved users, other disciplines or purchasers.

These last two points seemed to raise particular issues for nurses in implementing service improvement and will be explored in more depth in Chapter 3. Here the effective approaches are analysed.

Managing the change as a specific project

Managing a change as a specific project requires a systematic approach to planning and organising the change, often involving a project team. In some cases, an NDU steering group fulfilled part of this role; in others, a working group was set up to steer the innovation.

The effectiveness of this project management approach is reflected by the fact that several groups continued to meet beyond the implementation stage, to monitor progress and plan future development. The role played by the manager in shaping and pushing the project forward, and seeing it as open to modification where necessary, is linked to nurses' perception of management and their willingness to take on a management role alongside their clinical duties (*see* Chapter 3 for further discussion of nurses assuming a management role). A project management approach was evident in several of the units studied (*see* Box 4).

Box 4

The Maternity Unit had to plan and manage a major service change, following a period of sustained campaigning, at the same time as the unit moved to a new hospital. The link to a physical move may have fostered a more systematic project approach, but the manager also focused on the service users throughout the period of change and organised information exchange sessions with them during the run up to the change.

The Mental Health Unit faced difficult staff motivation problems. To solve these problems and map out a clear strategy to get staff on board, the clinical leader used the classic approach of involving them in project and teamwork activity. She was aware of the 'the low status of work...

Box 4 *cont'd*

staff have been a long time in their posts; clients are difficult; staff, especially the unqualified, are not involved in the high-level excitements of the change.' However, she herself had a remarkably systematic approach to planning the management of changes in this context; this was her strength.

The District Nursing Unit formed a project team to introduce a new scheme whereby district nurses would act as primary nurses in the hospital setting. The team tackled the involvement of general practitioners (GPs) and staff in this scheme in a planned way, organising meetings, a 'roadshow' and staff development activities. It then developed documentation to launch the scheme, such as revised drugsheets; these helped the nurses as well as the GPs, who had raised the issue during the roadshows.

As noted in Chapter 1, not all units had a clear strategy or plan, and they recognised that this could have helped them. Some units also experienced problems in clarifying the management role, which hindered the development of a clear project approach. An example of this is given in Box 5.

Box 5

In one unit the clinical leader was more senior than her counterparts in the other units. She was therefore relatively distant from the day-to-day aspects of the change and focused mainly on the broader issues and wider dissemination of the work. This meant that leadership and maintaining momentum at ward level were functions that sometimes seemed to fall through the net, resulting in patchy progress.

Using nurse expertise and power

Implicitly or explicitly, nurses' assessment of their own skills contributed greatly to planning the introduction of changes. The traditional view of nurses as 'handmaidens' to doctors, coping with all situations whatever the resources[6] and often going unheard as a group, militates against explicitly defining and using nurse expertise and power. The value of explicitly incorporating nurses' skills and power into the change process, however, was clear in several cases (*see* Box 6). A key aspect of their expertise is their intimate knowledge of what the clients, patients and their families want. Combined with their caring and personal skills, this is potentially a powerful resource in service improvement.

Box 6

In establishing the nurse-led Anorexia Unit, the clinical leader was clear about the skills that nurses have: a good knowledge of the client group; flexibility and creativity; an ability to get to know patients and talk to them in their language; and a capacity to identify a variety of success indicators for patients. For anorectics, for example, nurses may decide to help some patients to live with their condition, rather than aim for a 'cure'. They are frequently in a position of teaching junior doctors, and they have 'human' knowledge which motivates them to stay around to see the effect of treatment. The nurse manager took on the difficult process of establishing the nurse-led unit by making these skills explicit and using them to underpin the changed values of the new unit.

In the District Nursing Unit the staff were very aware of their positive reputation among GPs and in the hospital, and of the varied and highly developed skill base of their community practice. They used this to support a change which involved taking on primary nursing inside the hospital. The confidence this awareness brought them was noticeable; they were a capable, strong group with a clear programme of action for patients, and so were taken seriously. This impact is still evident as they continue extending their role by taking on nurse prescribing and nursing beds.

The Maternity Unit drew on the traditions and skills of midwifery and made these skills explicit. The staff also made it clear that they know what women want and the problems they face in maternity care. In this case, the knowledge was formalised through a study of users' experiences.

The issues raised by these observations are explored in Chapter 3, where aspects of change management which seem specifically to concern the nursing profession are analysed.

Taking account of external factors

The relevant external factors for practice-level changes include:

- national health priorities and current debates on these priorities
- the needs and views not only of local patients, clients and other service users but also of non-users of the service
- the communities served by the unit and their characteristics (e.g., ethnic group and age profiles)
- the current and likely local resource constraints
- trust status and possible future changes
- the most likely purchasers and their priorities
- the decision makers, their priorities and how decisions are reached.

Nurse managers in the units studied worked with these issues in different ways, both wading into the tide of events and seeking allies outside the unit, notably the King's Fund itself occasionally. Some units were able to use their own reputation and expertise to muster support from experts in their particular field at national level. In other cases, however, units found that national interest in their work did not create the necessary support at the trust management level, and support therefore had to be actively encouraged by ensuring that the service development was known about locally.

In general, the units were working within a context of negative external factors, such as cost reduction and the increasingly fragmented pattern of nurses' hours and shifts. These issues were commented on by operational staff, but some nurse managers or clinical leaders did not explicitly link them to the changes being implemented. This gave staff the impression that the day-to-day pressures on them were not being taken on board.

The issue of links with purchasers emerged as a key factor. Some units established strong links with purchasers, in one case with both the District Health Authority and the GP fundholders, who were invited to visit the unit. Here, the clinical leader fostered dialogue with purchasers about their needs, and reported that 'their reaction has been positive.' Elsewhere, staff made several references to a lack of clarity on the purchasers' role locally, and where no links were made it sometimes proved much more difficult to sustain positive changes.

The examples given in Box 7 illustrate cases where the changes introduced were in tune with specific external factors.

Box 7

A number of external factors contributed to the successful campaign to retain the Maternity Unit. These included: well-organised and vocal local campaigning groups; an approaching general election; and the national maternity review, 'Changing childbirth', which promoted a model based on greater choice for women. Midwives worked *with the grain* of these external factors, and actively campaigned themselves for the Maternity Unit to remain open. The clinical leader commented that: 'The public saw the Acute Service Review as a decision and didn't think it could be overturned. It [our leafleting] was trying to spur on a bit of impetus. Once the public got hold of it the momentum was retained. The local press was very good, very supportive. The public were very keen to see the unit established and successful.' This approach of campaigning jointly with users has continued to be a vital part of the team's work.

The Health Visitor Unit gained support for its projects by linking them to the government priorities published in *Vision for the Future,* and *Health of the Nation* and to the implications of community care, as well as to local concern about accident rates.

The efforts to establish the Anorexia Unit benefited from the prevailing public concern about anorexia. However, the clinical leader considered that the most important factor was the favourable market environment. The unit provides a greater range of services and more choice for patients. In spite of enormous difficulties in setting it up, she is convinced that without this favourable environment the unit would not have been established and that it will now grow and thrive.

Information exchange with stakeholders

Any change involves different groups of people and individuals affected by the change. The first task is to identify the key people, the *stakeholders*, and to work with them. The term 'stakeholders' refers to anyone with an interest in the organisation, such as relatives, local community groups (including women's associations and ethnic minority groups), staff at all levels and from different disciplines, managers in provider units, purchasers, professional bodies, education providers and voluntary organisations. The list may be a long one. The stakeholders most involved in the units studied were the consultants or GPs, patients/users and relevant nursing and other staff. Those least involved (sometimes quite unknown) were the purchasers. In the middle ground were the more senior managers of the trusts; their involvement is explored in Chapter 3, where the links between clinical leaders and the broader management issues in their organisations are discussed.

Stakeholders come to the situation with different views, different powers and different approaches to judging the success of the service improvement. The units managed their stakeholder relationships in a variety of ways.

The steering groups that each NDU formally sets up are one example of a mechanism to bring together the key people with an interest in the service, which elsewhere takes the form of a project team or working group. It is important to involve not only those who at the outset show support for the innovations, but also those who are not initially 'on board'. One manager, reviewing the failure to embed new ideas once key individuals had left, felt that she and her team had been too 'precious' in involving only their supporters. 'We should have had some people who would have asked us some sticky tricky questions,' she commented. While managing such groups is sometimes problematic, the lack of dialogue with key stakeholders seems to lead to greater difficulties once the implementation of the service improvement begins.

To highlight how the units liaised with stakeholders and which approaches were most and least successful in fostering the changes, the following discussion focuses on purchasers, service users and doctors.

Purchasers

The Maternity Unit was unusual in having strong links with the purchasers (the District Health Authority and the GP fundholders, as noted earlier). This unit used its expertise to 'market' its services actively. The midwives' intimate knowledge of what women want was formalised through a study of users' experiences. (This is in line with the research conducted by Pettigrew and his colleagues[7] on receptive contexts for change in the NHS, where coherence of policy, substantiated by relevant data, emerged as an important factor in successful innovation.)

Where links with purchasers were weak or absent, there was less chance of embedding improvements over the long term. (Embedding change is examined in Chapter 4.)

Service users

Users have the biggest stake in the service and any changes to it. Successful innovators actively encouraged service users to develop their power, in a way that went beyond the rhetoric of the 'customer', and took account of the complexities involved in empowering powerless groups and of staff giving up some professional power.

A clinical leader commented: 'Another thing we have learned is the power of the women: they do not realise how much power they have. They are very, very powerful. Unfortunately, because they don't realise their power, it tends to be the GP that holds a lot of the power. So working with the women, we can instil in them a sense of ownership.' Other staff were aiming to relinquish power. One of them said: 'You have to be prepared to change your practice completely, the base of professional knowledge is incomplete, you may be misinformed. What you know may be based on inaccurate information.'

Spending time with service users was seen as vital to empowering them and improving the nurses' understanding of their needs. This was not an easy task. One nurse commented: 'You can have as much time as you like with the patients – I'm used to working fast – it's hard to slow down.'

Service innovation involved actively changing the relationships between staff and service users. There are a number of ways in which users can participate in decisions affecting the service. Figure 2 lists these ways in the form of a continuum from the traditional mode to the empowered mode of user participation.

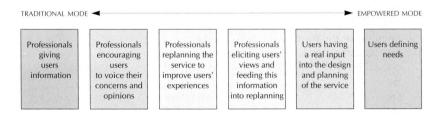

TRADITIONAL MODE ◀—————————————————————————▶ EMPOWERED MODE

| Professionals giving users information | Professionals encouraging users to voice their concerns and opinions | Professionals replanning the service to improve users' experiences | Professionals eliciting users' views and feeding this information into replanning | Users having a real input into the design and planning of the service | Users defining needs |

Figure 2: *Traditional and empowered modes of user participation*

To enable the least powerful members of communities, those traditionally without a 'voice', to have a real input into service planning and to define their own needs, professionals have found that they have to rethink their method of work, as well as the values and beliefs underlying it. All the units visited had explored a variety of ways of involving users, including the challenging approach of transferring power to users. It was particularly striking that the units working predominantly with women or with Black communities had taken this approach and that the values underlying their methods of work were usually explicitly voiced.

Doctors

Nurse leaders were most familiar with 'managing' different kinds of relationships with consultants, doctors and GPs. As with relationships with service users, here too the agenda was often, openly or implicitly, about redistributing power. Some changes which expanded the nurses' role reduced the workload for doctors and suited the doctors' interests. Building this partnership is a continuous and paradoxical process: nurses in the same unit, and sometimes the same nurses, have had contradictory experiences. This illustrates the need for more contact and discussion between stakeholders about changes in order to identify and deal with their different perceptions of the same issue. Change can act as a kind of X-ray on the work, showing up, often for the first time, the differences and problems between groups and individuals, and uncovering previously hidden disparities in power. Examples of working with stakeholders are given in Box 8.

Box 8

The consultant in the Maternity Unit had, in the past, been very pressured; he used to 'run from room to room' to see the patients. The ward is now a tranquil place where many of the consultants' duties are being undertaken by the midwives. The consultant also wanted to maintain the obstetric service, which required the Maternity Unit remaining open. The midwife-led option was a way of ensuring this. The clinical leader is aware, however, that consultants in the midwife-led unit may feel isolated and keeps them well informed of the issues midwives are facing.

Box 8 *cont'd*

The clinical leader of another unit emphasised how supportive the consultant was: 'We are very lucky; other nurses don't have supportive consultants... We have good collaboration with medical colleagues. They do respect us.' But she also reported that the consultant had said 'it's nice to have a nurse there – to help me'; she was adamant that 'we're not there for him, but for the patients.' Another consultant wanted to 'sneak in' an extra patient, saying he could do the treatment on a couch, to which the clinical leader replied: 'Don't tell me how to care for my patients.' She commented later: 'I'm far more assertive than I was before. I wish he'd understand that we're the only ones to understand the workload. He still hasn't changed. He gets a bit better, then he slides back.'

One of the major changes nurses commented on was that they were no longer the 'handmaidens' of the doctors. For example, they viewed doctors' knowledge and midwives' knowledge as being on a par, with different kinds of expertise involved, midwives being seen as more expert in normal births and doctors having the necessary expertise for dealing with high-risk births. However, one doctor in a different unit, when asked about the nursing staff undertaking a broader range of treatment, was very positive about the changes and then said: 'Well, you can teach a monkey to do anything.' This surprising statement does not reflect respect between stakeholders or a sharing of professional expertise and responsibilities. The doctor had not recognised that the expansion of the nurses' role had changed the power relationship and he continued to take nurses' contributions to care for granted.

It was, not surprisingly, in the doctor/nurse relationships that gender emerged as a key factor in managing changes. This is so much taken for granted that nurses and doctors seldom comment on it, but to a large extent the combination of male/female and doctor/nurse dynamics underlies traditional perceptions of the nurse's role. There are now more men working as nurses and more women as consultants but, as noted earlier, in the cases studied all the consultants were men and all the clinical leaders but one were women. One clinical leader who had worked with two male consultants said that neither had treated her like a professional colleague; one had treated her like a daughter, while the other alternately bullied and flirted with her. To gain their co-operation in establishing a new nurse-led service, she had to find ways of working with these two powerful men which did not threaten her own professionalism.

The issue of gender and its relevance to nurse managers is discussed further in Chapter 3.

Summary

Successful innovators had undertaken an explicit analysis of their key stakeholders and identified the stakeholders' areas of interest and the criteria upon which they would judge the unit. These innovators were also aware of the gender and 'race'[8] issues involved and how they would affect (though not govern) stakeholders' interests and powers. This enabled them to practise what might be called 'stakeholder management': with a clear picture of the differing interests and powers involved, they worked with the stakeholders to help them contribute to and support the service improvement. Where innovators had *not* 'managed' key stakeholders, problems emerged.

This chapter has looked at ways of managing change that helped nurse managers achieve their aims, and has raised some of the difficulties which hindered them; this will be discussed further in Chapter 3.

In their study on organisational change, Moss Kanter, Stein and Jick[9] suggest that in the change process there are three main groups of participants:

- change strategists, who look at the connection between the organisation and its environment
- change implementers, who are responsible for the internal organisational implications of introducing changes
- change recipients, who are affected by the change and react to it.

The key issue here is that these roles need not be held by separate individuals, although there may be a difference in perspective. Nurses often feel that they are implementers and recipients, rarely strategists. However, those introducing change in the units studied have clearly acted as change strategists as well as implementers in that they recognised that successful service improvement involves the following steps:

1 Identify the key people whose support for the change is needed (stakeholders) and assess their interest in the improvement

2 Treat stakeholders as 'invisible' members of the team who are vital to the success of the project and therefore need to be kept informed and involved

3 Plan and organise ways of gathering data from and/or with stakeholders, taking account of gender and 'race' issues

4 Analyse and market the strengths of the project, especially nurses' skills and expert knowledge (particularly knowledge of service users and their needs) and identify any weaknesses in order to counteract them

5 Be pro-active in using external factors where they are relevant to the change by looking for opportunities and threats in the wider environment, outside the unit

6 Keep a firm focus on the overall aims of the change by working to an explicit strategic plan

7 Pursue the plan actively, ensuring that the key stakeholders, including purchasers and senior managers, understand the plan and are kept informed of its progress.

All these elements appear in general 'recipes' for managing change, but the case studies showed that they are both necessary and yet can be difficult to achieve at operational level for nurse managers. The key principles so far identified from the case studies all illustrate *the importance of adopting a strategic approach to achieving service improvement,* no matter how small the change may appear to be.

Chapter 3
Nurse managers and change

The experience of clinical leaders in the units studied was that to improve the service, they had actively to take on the *managerial* as well as the clinical role. Chapter 2 focused on ways of managing change strategically that could apply to a manager in any organisation. This chapter focuses on those issues raised in Chapter 2 which are specific to *nurse* managers:

- accepting and playing a visible managerial role in the organisation, as well as a clinical role
- conceptualising change as an organisational process, as well as a clinical improvement
- naming and 'publishing' what nurses do
- identifying the gender and 'race' issues involved, particularly where these are built into the structure of the organisation.

All these issues are closely connected, and are considered separately here only for the purposes of discussion.

Accepting and playing both a managerial and a clinical role

Senior trust managers were not very visible in the work undertaken by clinical leaders to introduce changes. Some nurse managers learned painfully that however focused they were on improving the clinical service offered to patients or clients, it was critically important to liaise with senior management, particularly when communication from management was patchy or non-existent and where key resources were involved.

A nurse manager needs to be visible to two groups of people: those inside the unit and those outside it. Traditionally, nurses have been more comfortable with visibility inside the unit, caring for patients and working with staff to support, motivate and develop them. In the case studies it appeared that those activities which removed nurses from their closeness to patients or clients and took them into negotiations within the larger institution were less familiar and less welcome, and often led to feelings of isolation, frustration and unwanted responsibility.

However, these external activities and involvement in the wider management context is essential in managing and embedding change successfully (*see* Chapter 4).

Some of the clinical leaders were extremely skilled at these negotiations, and everyone recognised that nurses need to develop these skills further. It was also striking that it often took some time for the nurse managers to realise the potential power they had to make changes. One of them said: 'As nurses you are not used to having power. As a clinical leader you do have power. I've seen this only recently; personally I'm more assertive than before.'

Management outwards

Reflecting on the difficulties she had faced in setting up a new unit, one clinical leader felt that she had not known enough about the wider management issues. She commented that nurses tend to look to themselves for solutions and that there is a temptation to focus on management inside, with unit staff, and not look outwards. She had wanted to focus on the clinical innovations, but to secure premises for the new unit she had to go to endless 'head-banging meetings.' She saw the battles over premises both as an indication of the lack of acceptance of a nurse-led unit and as part of the wider skirmishes between men in powerful positions, skirmishes in which she had to be involved. 'It's like Bosnia out there,' she said. She also discovered that the new unit had not been included in the application for trust status and had to make sure that it was. Two years of poor communication from managers to nurses and her own lack of knowledge about management agendas were among the main issues she cited as hindering progress in establishing the new unit.

Another unit, faced with moving to new premises, a merger and the renegotiation of roles, was unable to identify a nurse manager to manage these changes successfully and it is possible that the service improvements will not be made.

These examples demonstrate that knowledge about the wider managerial issues is essential for successful service improvement: knowing who makes what decisions, and engaging in what many nurses feel is outside their core task of developing clinical practice. Entering the managerial arena requires a considerable investment of time, energy and courage, and is particularly important where communication is poor.

Management inside

The case studies showed that nurse managers had a high degree of expertise in staff development and motivation. Examples of what had been done in this respect include:

- setting up an appraisal scheme that involved unqualified long-stay staff in setting their own development objectives
- being pro-active in resolving conflict between members of staff by arranging meetings based on forcefield analysis (*see* Appendix 2)
- arranging staff visits (in the Mental Health Unit, by both qualified and unqualified staff) to other units to compare practice and culture
- setting up an internal standards group to discuss and decide upon standards of good practice
- delegating decisions on how to carry out activities
- introducing a work-shadowing scheme to enable two groups of staff to get to know each others' work routines and demands, which included the involvement of night staff
- establishing reading groups to discuss current relevant literature and identify possible ways forward for the change
- arranging meetings aimed specifically at re-motivating staff following a period of drift.

In the last example, a new nurse manager who had previously been one of the staff was appointed. She said: 'I was not the most senior, not a popular choice. Some needed time to absorb it, some had to re-establish their position. I let things drift for a bit, I think that was needed, then involved staff in projects.' These projects included: business planning meetings involving all staff; meetings of G grade sisters, which helped them to be cohesive and support each other; and operational team representatives' meetings.

Three particularly difficult issues in internal staff management were identified in several cases: the confusion of roles where clinical leadership was separated from management; the paradoxical results of the expansion of the nurses' role; and the problems related to the induction of new staff.

The confusion of roles where clinical leadership was separated from management caused a lot of time and emotional energy to be wasted on clarifying roles, and prevented clear leadership. In one unit, the 'buzz' of the changes working well was lost when power issues and poorly defined roles led to uncertainty about the future of the project and because the nurse manager had not focused enough on the management agenda to ensure that the changes would continue.

The paradoxical results of the expansion of the nurses' role were evident in several units. In a number of cases, junior nurses felt that their role had become *less* challenging. When doctors were not around, a more senior or more experienced nurse on duty took on responsibility, preventing junior nurses from making decisions they would previously have made, sometimes in consultation with the more senior nurse.

One nurse said: 'You are treated as if you don't know very much, as it [the work] is so different. It is hard not to be able to make decisions – difficult to stamp your personality on anything.' Her work was in some ways becoming more complex and the clinical leader's recruitment policy was to take on experienced nurses in order to cope with this. However, the standardisation of treatment procedures was viewed as a reduction of individual discretion and made it *seem* more simplified to the staff involved. Another example was where a midwife commented that in the midwife-led unit her work carried less responsibility than had been the case in her previous, doctor-led workplace, as there was always a senior midwife on duty who took responsibility.

These examples demonstrate the need to ensure that less senior nurses do not lose the breadth and depth of responsibility they are used to carrying, and to avoid a tendency to 'de-skill' staff. Changes in treatment procedures and an increase in the responsibility of more senior nurses raise different staff training needs for consideration by nurse managers. It is also necessary to think in detail about the actual work activities which a new system will create for all levels of staff.

The induction of new staff, especially to the culture and practice approach of the unit, needs to be handled carefully. In a unit with a strong culture of excellence and attention to patient needs, the *culture* was embedded and everyone was clear about the standards expected, but new staff felt they needed more support in learning new procedures and in adapting to new ways of working with patients or clients. One new nurse commented: 'There is a massive amount to learn. They [existing staff] are so quick you have to ask to do things, and you don't learn the rarer procedures. The consultants don't like to be kept waiting so the quickest nurse does it. The girls [sic] who have done it before do it.' In this unit, the new culture introduced by the clinical leader involves nurses spending a lot of time talking to patients or clients.

A nurse transferred from another inpatient unit found it difficult to adjust to this: 'I find it hard to slow down. They [the existing staff] do spend longer. So hard to sit. I couldn't bear it. I want to get on but I *know* it's more important to sit and talk.'

In contrast, in another unit a new member of staff who referred to herself as 'the baby of the team' was given a new area of work to develop and present, specifically as a way of integrating her into a long-established team. She was sent on a 17-day course on HIV and AIDS and asked to prepare a presentation to the team on the advantages and disadvantages of antenatal testing. This was welcomed by everyone involved.

Management inside and outwards

In a discussion on the need for management outside as well as inside the unit, one skilled nurse manager was clear that her role included managing external relationships and inputting ideas without dictating how things should be done. For example, she would pass on external news to the staff and say: 'This is becoming an issue we might be forced to address.' This would enable them, she said, 'to start thinking of solutions.'

Conceptualising change as an organisational change process as well as a clinical improvement

Changes were most effective where managers viewed them as organisational as well as clinical changes. There appeared to be several factors involved in managing this process, including: leadership; the use of systematic models of change processes; communication; and the use of evaluation information. Examples of how units dealt with these factors are given in Boxes 9 to 12.

Box 9

LEADERSHIP

One clinical leader was described enthusiastically as someone who 'gave you a feeling that you are trusted to evolve your own ideas – where there were no sacred cows' and was able to 'weld a multi-disciplinary team together.' Another was described by her staff as 'having done wonders. The amazing high standard of care is due to her, everyone

---

Box 9 *cont'd*

takes it from her.' By contrast, in another unit the leadership was contested. One of the two contenders was described as 'having the gleam in the eye without the push.' What was described as 'collaborative leadership' concealed competition and a lack of clarity.

Box 10

USING SYSTEMATIC MODELS OF CHANGE PROCESSES

Some nurse managers deliberately used tools and theories of change processes to help them implement changes. In one unit a survey on morale was conducted by a personnel officer, and away-days were then used to plan how to improve morale using forcefield analysis (*see* Appendix 2). The use of power net analysis (*see* Appendix 2) enabled the nurse manager to identify 'supporters' and 'resisters' and ways of turning the resisters into what she called 'change bearers'. Her group of long-serving staff included some who were very resistant to and fearful of NDU status. One of them was given specific responsibility for seeing through the change of the use of a room for staff into one for residents, a micro change that could have caused staff resentment, particularly in an enclosed culture; giving her 'ownership' of the project led to a change in her attitude.

Another clinical leader who was moving to a new unit where, again, there were long-serving staff, and who had experience with managing changes, wanted to try out introducing some of the changes in a different environment. This time, she planned to allow for much more staff initiative and had sent up 'trial balloons', organised a roadshow with staff from another unit, and provided a lot of information to the staff in her new unit. She was using a more incremental approach, but recognised that she might not get full agreement.

Box 11

COMMUNICATION

In the case studies, this was always an area where staff at different levels held different views, the nurse managers thinking that they had communicated fully, but staff feeling uninformed. 'I haven't been told how it will work,' said one nurse about a new proposal. 'We'll be told about it. I have a feeling it is already planned.' Communication was vital with service users too. In commenting on a patient's feedback, a nurse wrote: 'She writes any queries she has. It prompts her to ask questions. We developed it in direct response to the audit which showed that patients did not receive all the information we thought we had given them.'

Box 12

USING EVALUATION INFORMATION

Where units were using feedback and formal audits to develop their service and practice, they recognised that they were in a process of continuous improvement with users. One unit set up a focus group of users to provide a more independent evaluation 'to test our perceptions' and control the tendency of staff to direct and exclude users through the use of jargon. The nurse manager explicitly linked this approach to achieving genuine improvements: 'We need to take users' comments seriously, work through and modify the project and process – and ultimately modify the service – to have cause and effect.' This contrasted with a more traditional research model where the separation of the research process had led to differences between researchers and practitioners.

The clinical leader of another unit was also very explicit about the need for an improvement model: 'A lot of our work is trying to improve on what people reflect to us are good qualities of our care, and also trying to improve on the bad things. We do quite a lot of perception studies, feedback from clients, a reunion group.' Interestingly, she commented that: 'Changes haven't been the result of formal evaluation, but have been the result of informal observation. I think that is what makes it difficult to recognise changes we have made.'

Naming and 'publishing' what nurses do

A key theme that emerged for nurse managers was the issue of naming and recognising their value. One clinical leader said: 'Nurses don't recognise their power: they accept a subservient role. Basic nursing skills are not valued, individual nurses are not valued: they are seen as interchangeable.' Another described the issue as: 'How to actually act; how to take responsibility to act within the role within which we are trained, and to respond to what our consumers are telling us. Having the confidence in our abilities to do that. That is one of the biggest lessons: that we are able to do it. We have our own capabilities, things that we can offer. That has enabled us to carry our practice forward. One of the biggest stumbling blocks for a lot of nursing professionals is that they haven't learned that awareness of their professional capabilities.'

There is a need for awareness of the scope and strengths of the nursing role and practice, as well as the confidence to use that awareness in working for change with the other stakeholders, who often have quite limited perceptions of the role of nurses in the organisational setting.

Interviewees in the case studies stressed that nurses need to 'identify what they do and learn to talk about it.' Robinson and Vaughan[11] also refer to the idea that nurses 'know more than they can tell' and to the lack of recognition of the intuitive knowledge they develop through their practice. One nurse manager commented that she was seen as an exception because she was able to articulate the reasons for a nurse-led service. She felt it was essential for all nurses to develop the confidence to make these strengths explicit and to view their 'human knowledge' as just as valuable as the doctors' 'technical knowledge'. She stressed the need 'to be able to write coherently, or to find someone who can.'

There were specific ways in which this was done in the units. The King's Fund focus on dissemination of good practice has encouraged people to try out many ways of 'publishing' nurses' activities and developments, from conferences to roadshows to writing care-maps. The term 'publishing' is used in preference to 'publicising' because it implies that making activities known is a positive move which brings some solidity and recognition to the work, whereas 'publicising' sometimes carries negative or superficial overtones and may seem too self-promoting.

It also emerged from the case studies that developing a national reputation for the work, while important, was no substitute for working

for recognition within the local community or within the hospital as a whole. Units found their work recognised and quoted in national fora and yet had to struggle for resources and recognition in their own trust or district. Clearly, this issue is also linked to the need to enter the management arena, as discussed earlier.

Both local and national level 'publishing' are encouraged by the King's Fund. The least 'publishing' activity undertaken has been within the units' own trust or locality. This perhaps raises issues of how women in particular see the value of making their achievements widely known and what they feel it is legitimate for them to do. One senior service manager, a woman, acknowledged that she should do more to 'market herself' and her nurses' activities, adding: 'I suppose that's a female thing, we'd rather just get on with the work.' This issue is closely related to 'coping management', which is discussed in Chapter 5.

It is also related to what Illich[12] calls 'vernacular values', which he contrasts with 'commodity values'. He views goods which are not for sale on the market as having 'vernacular value' and favours placing more emphasis on the area of social life which has vernacular rather than commodity value and less emphasis on those areas where market or commodity values operate. Although he does not link the concept of vernacular value to gender, it is evident that much of the work traditionally done by women has vernacular rather than commodity value (e.g., housework). This evaluation extends from women's unpaid work into their paid work, in particular into caring occupations such as nursing. Society's evaluation of women's work also influences women's *own* evaluation of their work. This may be another reason why female nurses find it difficult to 'publish' their work.

Within this context, the issue of intellectual property and copyright of innovation was raised in interviews during the case studies. Two views emerged:

- nursing practice is 'not derived from the market, its value cannot be costed, it is built out of personal experience' and information on innovation should therefore be shared freely across the NHS
- innovation has a value which can be of benefit to the innovating institution by copyrighting the ideas to ensure survival in a competitive environment.

Plans to 'publish' work do require a clear view to be taken on this issue.

Identifying the gender and 'race' issues involved

Throughout discussions in the units gender and 'race' implications of managing change were rarely raised explicitly. The predominance of women in nursing and that of men in medical posts, and the absence of black staff, were largely accepted unconsciously; the existence of lesbian and gay staff or service users and of staff with disabilities was not recognised. Some readers may indeed question the need to raise these issues here. However, where the changes involved a shift in role, and therefore in power, between nurses, doctors and service users, gender and 'race' issues were also involved. Analysing them may help nurse managers to identify sources of resistance and support for change much more clearly and to understand more fully the dynamics of the change process.

In the case studies there were a number of situations where gender or 'race' issues were relevant to the service improvement. Some of them were commented on by the people involved. The situations discussed here relate to: power shifts; domestic roles affecting work; women's influence on patients' experiences; individual diversity at work; and where silence prevailed.

Power shifts

In some cases, a shift in power in relation to the use of knowledge and skill was accompanied by a gender or 'race' shift. There was a shift in power where nurses took a leading role which in the cases studied meant a shift from men leading to women leading. Elsewhere, there was also a careful and thoughtful, though difficult, attempt to shift power in terms of whose knowledge was valued. Here the shift was accompanied by a shift from valuing the knowledge of white professionally qualified health workers to valuing that of black and ethnic minority patients and clients and less conventionally qualified health support workers. Examples of power shifts are given in Box 13.

Domestic roles affecting work

An example of where gender in relation to domestic roles influenced approaches at work is given in Box 14.

Box 13

In the Maternity Unit, where obstetrics has been a male-dominated, medically oriented speciality, the new working assumption is that the midwife is the expert in normal childbirth and will call in a consultant or registrar only if there are problems. Women are in charge and are seen as having the knowledge and skill to take a leading role. 'The whole thing has changed about. And it is a threat to some people. At first women were coming and expecting to see the doctor and would express disappointment. Now we notify them that their first visit will be with a midwife. She understands what she is coming for.' The male consultant, however, is still nominally in charge – 'My name appears at the top of the paper' – and currently likes to see every patient at least once. This will change, but will have to be acceptable to the GPs referring pregnant women.

In the Neighbourhood Healthcare Unit, 'race' issues were particularly important and tended to be bound up with gender issues. The lack of Bangladeshi staff in the unit was viewed as a limiting factor in the change strategy. There is currently only one Bangladeshi health visitor in the borough. In this situation the non-Bangladeshi health visitors had consciously to set aside their assumptions and even knowledge in order to listen to and learn about the Bangladeshi women they were trying to help. The Health Centre has appointed a Bangladeshi woman to a new post of Health Visitor Assistant, and the trust employs link workers and interpreters. There are still problems about defining the skills and experience needed for these posts, ensuring proper recognition and pay, and creating a structure for career development and access to training. There are also dilemmas about the dual identity required of 'representatives' of minority communities, who may lose their ability to speak for the communities if they become identified, by themselves and the communities, with the trust.

Box 14

The involvement of nurse managers in changes in one unit was made difficult by the assumption that they were free to attend meetings outside working hours to exchange information or develop their skills. This raised two problems: resentment, by partners who were also nurses,

---

Box 14 *cont'd*

about career progression; and childcare responsibilities. As in other professions, responsibility for organising childcare generally falls on the woman, even where the male partner does the childcare. In another unit, all members of a project team were mothers and they shared childcare.

Women's influence on patients' experiences

There were several cases where those interviewed considered that having a staff comprised entirely or mainly of women influenced the way that patients or clients were treated. Examples of this influence are given in Box 15.

Box 15

Having women in charge had an impact on the work itself and on the environment, which in several cases was noticeably more calm and relaxed, as well as on the more practical aspects such as toilet facilities. There was a continuing effort among nurses to secure choice for their patients or clients about mixed wards or mixed toilets, especially where space was at a premium. The influence of women generally resulted in a more user-related and 'low-tech' approach, compared with the male-influenced tendency to push for more 'high-tech' interventionist treatment. Where all the patients or clients were women this approach was particularly noticeable. One midwife commented that: 'Working with women makes it something special, we try and make it as nice as is possible', adding that if she herself ever gave birth she would like a female midwife.

Individual diversity at work

In some units, work relationships were influenced by personal issues of identity and power, as illustrated by the experiences described in Box 16.

Box 16

In the units visited, inter-professional relationships were more difficult in the cases of differences in age, gender and 'race' where these coincided with marked differences in approach to change management. Together, these factors produced major barriers to genuine dialogue. As Moss Kanter[13,14] observed in her research, the isolated, highly visible and lone representative of any minority experiences conflicting pressures to over-achieve, overwork and take on the attributes of the majority to gain acceptance and recognition, or to exaggerate the attributes of his/her own group which the majority may value. This is analogous to nurses 'coping' in the face of impossible demands and resources in order to gain approval and perhaps a measure of protection.

Silence

As noted earlier, the absence of black staff was largely accepted unconsciously, while the existence of staff with disabilities and of lesbian and gay staff, patients or clients was not recognised. While this may reflect the national situation in the NHS, it clearly requires action at every level, in particular to meet the diverse needs of service users and promote a positive culture for all groups. The observations made during the study are outlined in Box 17.

Box 17

With one or two exceptions, there was a significant absence of black staff in the units visited. However, none of the case study visits was made during night shifts (and not all units involved carried out night-time services), and there may have been black staff on night duty. If so, this would be an example of marginal employment. With few exceptions, the absence of black staff was not commented on by interviewees. There was a similar silence on the needs of lesbian and gay patients or clients and on issues for staff who are lesbian, gay or disabled.

Summary

The discussion of who is 'absent' and who it 'present' will be taken up again in Chapter 5. Some of the issues raised in this chapter are primarily for individual nurse managers to consider and analyse in order to set development goals for themselves or in consultation with their supervisors. But the wider issues raised about the links between nursing, management, gender, 'race' and other organisational issues also need to be considered by those in the profession who are developing the nurse role overall, as well as the training and education this requires. They also pose a clear challenge to trust management in developing organisational structures and culture.

The conclusion from the case studies is that, for successful change in service provision, nurses need to recognise and develop their management role. This requires:

- giving constant consideration to the *organisational aspects* of the change, as well as the clinical elements which are naturally their first focus
- focusing on *managing outwards* as well as inside their unit
- identifying their strengths and *publishing the achievements* of their work in their own institution (and more widely, if possible)
- bringing into their management practice the *hidden or absent dimensions* relating to gender, 'race', disability and sexuality when developing service improvements.

This chapter looks at the dilemmas and paradoxes raised by service improvement, which become evident when trying to make changes 'stick' or to overcome major barriers. From the case studies, it is clear that to be pro-active rather than simply responding to events, change strategists need to:

- consider how best to *embed* successful changes so that they last into the future, whatever happens to the people originally involved (this is to avoid the problem identified by Goodman and Dean:[15] 'Change has been successfully introduced, some benefits appeared; but over time the majority of programs had become deinstitutionalised.')
- recognise and exploit unplanned opportunities to act *creatively* and quickly to achieve the desired change, as well as planning change systematically.

Embedding change

Embedding involves managing the paradox between making a change 'stick' so that it lasts (e.g., after the departure of key staff or beyond the next wave of changes) and at the same time making sure that the organisation is not 'stuck', either tied down in inflexible procedures or people feeling they cannot further improve the service. The ways nurse managers were dealing with this tension fell broadly into two kinds of approach: *procedural* and *cultural*. Most tended to rely on one or the other, but the strongest sense of embedded change came from projects where *both approaches* were used.

This dual approach is important since it could be easy to criticise the procedural approach as 'bureaucratic' and representing 'paper policy'. However, in an organisational bureaucracy such as that which prevails in much of the public sector in Britain, so-called bureaucratic or procedural approaches are essential if the system is to work well. The cultural 'people-based' approach is necessary, but some managers discovered that without procedural embedding in the structures of the organisation, changes could disappear when key people moved on.

This was an important insight.

Procedural approach

Examples of a procedural approach in the case studies included:

- using job descriptions to incorporate new or re-specified tasks or responsibilities
- building the changes into purchaser's service specifications
- developing review systems to monitor progress and provide measurable indicators of change
- including and acknowledging innovation in formal documents such as business plans, trust annual reports and purchaser/commissioner documents
- providing systematic training for staff, including induction into both the task and process aspects of the changes
- developing documentation for changed procedures or duties.

In one unit, a new treatment management approach was the basis of a new computerised system and became a lasting manifestation of the change. Although people took time to get used to using it, within a few months nurses were talking positively about how much it helped them. The information was also used as a measure of volume of work and therefore of staffing needs, giving the nurse manager solid information to feed into budget discussions and bids for more staff.

Documentation was introduced for system changes. For example, case management forms are now being used to document patient progress, and they will probably continue to be used since documentation is especially prone to an 'inertia effect'. Other units had ensured their work was included within the trust business plan, setting out intentions to continue with or extend the service improvement.

A procedural approach to embedding service changes helps manage the following paradoxes:

What people do	vs	what people say
Individual leading change	vs	organisational culture
Building trust in individuals	vs	building change into the structure of the organisation

Cultural approach

Examples of a cultural approach in the case studies included:

- team-building to focus staff attention on the task and its impact on patients, and to develop their pride in and commitment to the changes
- building a 'critical mass' of opinion or skills to carry through the changes and support them over time
- fostering critical dialogue between stakeholders to reflect on and continuously develop of the service (e.g., through joint audit, liaison groups or ways of service user involvement)
- ensuring a constant acting out and practice of the new work or role to make it an established part of the organisational culture, so that doing otherwise became impossible.

In one case, a strong culture of excellent practice was embedded through deliberate team-building as a result of targeted recruitment, and through the personal leadership of the clinical leader. It was reinforced by the high standards required by consultants. Although some procedural elements were used, staff induction and systematic on-job training were missing, leading to the danger that the careful team-building would be in vain if the most experienced staff were unable to share their skills and knowledge.

In another case, this team-building approach was used with great success in terms of getting the unit's initiatives going and creating 'a great buzz' in a culture of shared social values. However, no attention was paid to involving the trust in the 'buzz', to procedural elements such as job descriptions or to purchaser specifications. The departure of key staff has resulted in the dissipation of the unit and the loss of much of the new approach it pioneered.

In a unit which had adopted a procedural approach, the close liaison with doctors was clear but that with ward nurses was much more patchy. The team-building was harder with this group of long-serving staff and had also been tackled over a relatively long timescale, leading to a loss of belief in the change among ward staff. Another unit experienced similar difficulties. It focused mainly on procedural aspects and intended to develop a critical mass of skills, but poorly defined management procedures and the lack of a genuine dialogue between stakeholders during the project undermined the chances of the change surviving the move of the unit to another hospital.

A cultural approach to embedding service changes helps manage the following paradoxes:

Individual vision	vs	organisational action
Individual development/thinking	vs	critical dialogue
Nurse-led change	vs	stakeholder-developed change
Front-line level information (providers)	vs	macro research-level information (purchasers)

Managing this last paradox is particularly important when nurses are working to a contract, where services are specified within the purchaser/provider relationship. Without input to the purchasers and dialogue with them, service development risks losing the richness of 'bottom-up' change. The Neighbourhood Healthcare Unit illustrated the power of working directly with users and purchasers, demonstrating the benefits of this to all stakeholders. This required team commitment to real involvement with users and to personal learning within the project, beyond pre-determined professional knowledge. The long timescale necessary to influence purchaser specifications also needed recognition.

Nurse managers who used both types of embedding approach carried through the service improvement successfully and gained personal satisfaction that it would be long-lasting despite the difficulties of achieving it. The positive strategies adopted by these nurse managers are listed in Box 18.

Box 18

The positive embedding strategies adopted by nurse managers in the units studied included:

- developing stakeholder commitment and involvement, and continuing this in formal mechanisms for dialogue with doctors, users, nurses and purchasers
- feeding information about service improvements into discussions with purchasers about future provision through contracts
- building nurse expertise in their expanded roles and building their confidence as a team

---

Box 18 *cont'd*

- linking specific jobs and services to government policy objectives (e.g, 'Health of the Nation' targets)
- organising careful inter-professional audit to develop services, evaluate success and continue to improve
- documenting user satisfaction with the changed service by conducting surveys, soliciting feedback at all times and using this information to modify the service as necessary
- contributing through the changed service to the trust's need to provide cost-effective services
- working closely with service users, actively encouraging a value-driven approach to their care
- using a systematic approach to staff development, linked to projects with measurable results for patient care
- reporting back on projects publicly within the hospital
- focusing staff development work on building a team in an enclosed and restricted environment
- paying attention to overcoming resistance by building staff 'ownership' of initiatives by involving them in responsibility for aspects of the change
- ensuring that new documentation had the support of key stakeholders.

Using creativity in managing change

Balancing the strategic plan with 'crafting strategy' (recognising opportunities that emerge during the change process and making creative use of them) is a key aspect of managing change that was evident in varying degrees in the cases studied.

Mintzberg[16] contrasts 'crafting strategy' with a 'rational planning' approach. He uses the analogy of a potter working with clay: 'Her mind is on the clay but she is also aware of sitting between her past experiences and her future prospects. She knows exactly what has and has not worked for her in the past. She has an intimate knowledge of her work, her capabilities, and her markets. As a craftsman [sic] she senses rather than analyses these things: her knowledge is "tacit"...

The clay sticks to the rolling pin, and a round form appears. Why not make a cylindrical vase? One idea leads to another, until a new pattern forms. Action has driven thinking: a strategy has *emerged*'. [Italics added]

Strategy is not all systematic planning. It can also include positively exploiting opportunities that emerge. Both planning and opportunism[17] are needed to cope with the dynamic circumstances nurse managers are usually facing. This is increasingly necessary to achieve lasting improvements in a fast-changing environment such as the health service.

Creativity also means thinking about new ways to do things, perhaps if resources are not available when needed or are inappropriate. The question some of the units were faced with was: How else can we do this? It is useful to return to this question again and again, especially when progress seems to be blocked or it becomes necessary to do something without incurring extra cost. Examples of the creative use of opportunities in the cases studied include:

- an anti-closure campaign launched by midwives
- the development of a telephone advice line to help outpatients
- completely new health visitor practices, including setting up community groups and organising campaigns
- a trip to the USA for training and advice on case management
- the use of an unplanned situation (when a distressed patient needed help) to develop the idea of primary nursing for district nurses in the hospital
- an acceptance of different treatment outcomes for anorectic patients which did not focus only on prescribed cures
- the use of staff development projects to provide service improvements for mental health patients
- persuading information technology staff to treat the service improvement as a pilot project and develop a computerised system free of charge.

Summary

Managing paradoxes is an inescapable part of public sector management The cases demonstrated a number of ways of embedding change that help to chart a course through these paradoxes. The constancy of change, especially in the external environment, also requires a nurse manager to take chances, create opportunities and use resources fully.

When planning or considering a service improvement, it is important *at the outset* to assess approaches for embedding the change. The main issues to consider are:

- the way in which the *type of service improvement* may itself suggest a procedural or cultural approach
- the need to build on this and consider *what gaps* might be left to be filled
- the value of recognising and *working with strengths in personal management style* (e.g., in organising groups of stakeholders) and at the same time recognising areas needing more attention (e.g., in applying a procedural approach to embedding change, such as gaining formal acknowledgement from trust managers)
- working with stakeholders to *develop new ways*, not mentioned in this study, to embed changes
- the importance of a *partnership* relationship with the purchaser.

It is becoming increasingly important to ask, throughout the change process: *How else* could we do this? Seeking answers to this question stimulates creativity and positive response to opportunities which are vital elements of a strategic management repertoire.

Chapter 5
The strategic shift for nurses

The purpose of this chapter is to identify ways in which nurse managers can apply a strategic approach to service improvement. Drawing on observations in the units studied, the discussion looks at successful approaches to providing a better experience for patients or clients and how these approaches differed from 'coping management'. It also examines some of the assumptions underlying the organisation of healthcare work which may make strategic approaches to management difficult for nurses.

Some of these assumptions, such as the division of labour between nurses and doctors, were being challenged in productive ways in the units visited, but others, such as 'male' and 'female' patterns of work, went unmentioned and unchallenged. When assumptions remain unexamined, they can contribute to what is termed the 'organisational neglect' of nursing and make it more difficult for nurse managers to change the structures of service delivery. This chapter offers specific suggestions on how to uncover and challenge such assumptions.

The chapter concludes with a summary of what was learned from the case studies about the ways in which nurse managers can shift to a strategic focus and what their organisations should do to support them.

From 'coping management' to strategic management

Strategic approaches used in the case studies

In conducting the case studies, there seemed initially to be a great diversity in the situations, service improvements and approaches used to manage the changes. Later, however, it became clear that similar approaches and issues were evident in all eight cases. The approaches which nurse managers found successful were:

- acting in a way which was explicitly managerial, engaging with organisational as well as clinical issues

- recognising the need for strategic approaches to apparently minor changes, since they are connected to broader issues, and assessing the impact of macro-level change on actual work practices
- taking a sustained approach to embedding changes, using a combination of procedural and cultural approaches (i.e., thinking through both ways of making change 'stick' by introducing new procedures or specifications, as well as different ways of working with people)
- developing links with purchasers and their information sources at the practitioner level (this is still a very new area for most nurses)
- using the power nurses have when they are aware of their expertise and make managers and other professionals aware of it
- acting out the practice they require of their staff and building the team culture to support it
- thinking beyond immediate concerns, experimenting, linking theory and practice, and using models which conceptualise social and organisational change.

'Coping management'

In her work on management styles in nursing, Davies[18] identified the style she terms 'coping management'. She defines a 'coping' manager as one who focuses on 'the immediate work to be done and on the means by which it can be accomplished within existing resources.' It is a 'firefighting approach to management that is accompanied by a strong personal commitment to the task, a weak sense of status and position, and a willingness, sometimes quite literally on the part of the manager, to "roll up the sleeves" and get on with whatever needs to be done'.

This is an image which many of the nurses identified with strongly. Indeed, there is an historical perception of nurses as 'doers' which has traditionally been reinforced by both junior and senior staff valuing those who do 'roll up their sleeves'.

Davies argues that coping management arises from the structures and conditions under which nurses work, in which gender plays an important role as 90 per cent of nurses are women. She describes the 'constant juggle to achieve cover'[19] which she says is attributable to:

- the lack of recognition of the gender issues involved in a career structure that rewards a full-time continuous work pattern, even where most staff have domestic and family roles requiring a different pattern

- the fact that, because of their domestic roles, a third of nurses work part-time, resulting in lower pay and grading, unsociable hours and night work and requiring complex shift patterns
- the use of bank nurses and, in the past, student nurses to cover the work required.

These complex work patterns need detailed supervision, which makes strategic management more difficult. In addition, the complexity of these internal management arrangements makes it difficult for nurses to make them intelligible to others. This contributes to the problem of defining what nurses do (*see* Chapter 3).

All these factors reinforce the low status of nursing compared with medical work, and the 'organisational neglect' of nursing. Davies describes how they lead to the coping style of management and of getting things done without complaint, which in itself reinforces organisational neglect. She also draws attention to the ways in which nursing is 'a female-gendered and devalued activity' and to the lack of support for the development of a knowledge base for nursing compared with medical knowledge. (*See* Chapter 3; the King's Fund Nursing Developments Programme was set up to make explicit and extend this knowledge base).

'Coping management' is often interpreted as a 'feminine' way of managing. However, Davies shows that, rather than being a 'feminine attribute', it is a consequence of two factors:

- the workplace is structured around working patterns set by men to fit society's norms of 'male' work, which do not take account of domestic responsibilities
- nurses have difficulty in 'naming' what they do, which militates against developing the knowledge base and challenging the 'organisational neglect' of nursing.

Thus, some of the barriers to developing a strategic perspective to management, rather than just 'coping', are *organisational rather than personal*. This suggests that it is *the infrastructure of organisations themselves that needs changing.*

From personal to organisational learning: surfacing assumptions

Tackling the infrastructure of an organisation requires discussion and dialogue through what is known as *organisational learning*. This involves encouraging people at all levels in the organisation to uncover and discuss underlying assumptions: assumptions about work, roles, knowledge, skills, values and who holds power. The units studied had uncovered and challenged a number deeply held assumptions.

Areas where assumptions were challenged

These areas included:

- the division of labour between doctors and nurses
- the role of patients and clients in defining their own goals and needs
- the role of professional knowledge compared with the experience of patients or clients
- the use of 'high-tech' versus 'low-tech' approaches to care
- the causes of ill health
- who is leading care in the context of the shift to community care
- the value given to nurses' knowledge.

Challenging the unspoken assumptions in these areas required what Weil[20] calls 'significant learning', whereby staff have to 'relinquish and transform deeply rooted attitudes, assumptions and beliefs'. In most of the units, 'significant learning' has been accomplished across the professions and through constructive dialogue and consensus (although this may be because it serves particular stakeholder interests).

'Din' and 'silence'

Other ways of uncovering underlying assumptions include identifying who is present and who is absent (as discussed in Chapter 3), where there is 'din' and where there is 'silence', and what it is legitimate or not legitimate[21] to talk about. Pettigrew and his colleagues[22] see legitimacy as 'a central concept linking political and cultural analyses [and] essential to the understanding of continuity and change ... the mechanisms used to legitimate and delegitimate particular ideas ... are crucial.'

Earlier chapters commented on who was overwhelmingly and appropriately present for nurse managers carrying out change, such as the patients or clients and doctors, and on notable absences, such as purchasers and black nurses.

'Din' and 'silence' are useful concepts to sum up what everyone is talking about in an organisation and what no one is talking about. They offer a way of measuring what is seen as important, what is seen as legitimate and what people are rewarded for in that organisation. In the case studies it was observed that:

- the 'din' in the units concerned excellent practice in nursing
- there was relative silence about cost pressures and trust concerns
- there was relative silence about power and gender, power and 'race', lesbian and gay nurses, doctors and patients or clients, and staff with disabilities.

The effect of these silences and absences may include:

- limited capacity of a team or unit to recognise the needs of specific service users (e.g., black or lesbian users)
- the absence of staff with the relevant knowledge and experience (e.g, managerial and operational staff from these groups)
- failure to involve major stakeholders in efforts to embed service improvements.

The effect of the 'din' can be the assumption that everyone agrees on a change, and the exclusion of related issues of costs, power and the broader trust agenda from discussion and planning at team level. Both effects can produce major problems in achieving service improvements (*see* Chapter 3).

'*Verbal leakage*'

Another way of uncovering assumptions is for nurse managers to listen carefully to themselves and others. People can learn a rhetoric, such as the rhetoric of 'involvement' of 'customers', of 'the community', of 'empowering' junior staff and of 'high-quality' services. For real organisational learning to take place, this rhetoric needs to be transformed into action. People directly involved will know if this has happened from their daily experience. Listeners can sometimes be alerted to whether something is rhetorical or real by what may be called 'verbal leakage', words which slip out that indicate what a person *really* thinks and therefore how he or she might behave. Examples of verbal leakage encountered in the case studies are given in Box 19.

> **Box 19**
> Examples of verbal leakage from the case studies included (italics added):
>
> - talking persuasively about how to support and involve members of the community in designing services, but saying: 'The *trick* is the support has to be *genuine*.' (Note the paradox)
> - being enthusiastic about staff empowerment, but talking about *my* school nurses, *my* health visitors, *my* district nurses'
> - saying, in a discussion about valuing the extended nurse role: 'But you can teach a monkey to do anything' (*see* Chapter 2).

Thus, to uncover assumptions, it is important that nurse managers listen to themselves and others, observe actions, and share what they hear and see. In the case studies, *some deeply held assumptions about power were challenged and changed in ways which improved services for patients or clients. Other assumptions were not uncovered but could have been, with positive results.*

We turn now to summarising how organisations and nurse managers can take action to foster organisational learning and develop their own strategic focus for achieving service improvements.

Shifting to a strategic focus

Writers in many fields of management have tried to define the term 'strategic', but there is little agreement except that it is a multi-faceted rather than single concept. Having a strategic focus means both having a particular attitude, a set of tools and techniques, and a process for managing. The suggestions for strategic action given here embrace all these and offer learning from the case studies as a starting point for further development and learning in readers' own organisations.

The organisation

Analysis of the cases showed how the underlying structuring of organisations could obstruct or work against nurses taking strategic approaches. In order to tackle this, organisations should consider:

- their *reward systems*, both formally (in terms of the impact of pay structures) and informally (how their culture recognises, for example, involvement in projects)

- creating *stable, recognised and permanent arrangements* for flexible employment, rather than using piecemeal and casual employment practices
- *presence and absence*, in terms of the diversity of all types and grades of staff and the organisation's consequent ability to identify and work positively with a diversity of patients or clients
- their *culture with regard to nursing and nurses* and their willingness to develop, include and promote nurses as partners, esteemed as highly as other professionals in the organisation.

Nurse managers

While the organisational issues are important for long-term changes, nurse managers can still pursue a strategic focus themselves. In the case studies, nurse managers not only took action to achieve better services but also challenged existing thinking. Drawing from their experiences, nurse managers intent upon improving services should think beyond 'coping' and take a strategic approach.

A STRATEGIC APPROACH

Think absence	Who is not involved but should be?
Think presence	Who is involved and is this explicit?
Think big	Everything connects to the 'big' issues (health needs, equity, the purchaser/ provider split, community care, power, authority and knowledge).
Think of the end	What is the situation you want to end up with?
Think of patients and clients	What decisions can they take? *What information do they need?*
Think of the outside	The external environment to the unit has a major impact.
Think of the inside	How will you take staff along with you?
Think skills	Explicit communication of what nurses do and know.
Think organisation	How can the whole trust benefit from the change and learn from your experience?
Think long term	What will help the change last and become embedded ?
Think practical	Recognise what you can and cannot do something about.
Think creative	How else could issues be tackled? What are your opportunities?
Think 'public'	Publish and 'market' the achievements of the team.
Think power	Who has it and who should have it? Who will support you and who oppose you?

Appendix I
Case studies of service improvement

Each case profile is presented, giving a summary of:

- the service improvement on which the unit was working
- the change(s) the unit had to make
- the 'triggers' for the change to happen
- how the change was introduced.

Case 1

THE MENTAL HEALTH UNIT offers very long-stay residential care for individuals with continuing mental health needs. The average length of stay is 42 years. The residents are described in the Annual Report as 'highly dependent and disturbed individuals'. Other residents living in flats on the site are actively resistant to resettlement outside the hospital; their average length of stay is 35 years. All the residents are male. Many of the staff have also been in the unit for a long time.

What was the service improvement?

There was low morale among existing staff, and it was difficult to attract new staff. It had been seen as a low-status area of work and, in the past, low-performing staff had been moved to this ward. It is a contracting area of work; older residents have died, and staff who had known them for years suffered distress. There is also uncertainty about who the new purchasers for this service will be. It is an example of a workplace with long, close working relationships among a small number of staff where small issues can get magnified. The ward manager wanted to develop ways to raise and maintain morale so that people worked positively together in these rather enclosed, long-enduring conditions and residents received good care. The work needs special staff with high motivation. The clinical leader aimed 'to increase openness and collaboration between staff, and to reduce negative staff interactions' in order to improve the service.

What was the change?

The method used to achieve change focused on staff development through a range of projects. The aim was to broaden staff members' perception of their input into the care received by patients and to raise professional standards. Five projects were identified as vehicles for staff development:

- *clinical supervision*
- *staff development system* (including personal and professional profiles and staff appraisal)
- *information technology* (piloting the computerisation of patient information and care plans and producing a staff magazine for the whole Rehabilitation Unit)
- *quality initiatives* (including standard setting and auditing, with the active involvement of users and relatives)
- *research-based care planning* (to question established nursing practice, involving research awareness and a database of resources, linked to goal planning for individual patients).

What were the triggers for change?

The opportunity to become an NDU crystallised ideas for improvement that the clinical leader was already considering. The need was initially identified with a selected group of staff (Annual Report 1993). A survey of morale conducted by the personnel manager found that unqualified staff felt they were not getting enough feedback from qualified staff, and that there was a lot of petty friction and ill feeling.

How was the change introduced?

An informal group consisting of the clinical leader, the ward manager, the rehabilitation specialist and two project nurses began meeting to carry through the changes that were formalised in a hurried application to the King's Fund. To meet the deadline meant there was little staff involvement, producing stresses for both the clinical leader and the staff, who viewed the introduction of the projects as 'too fast to start with'. Subsequently, the clinical leader took a systematic approach, believing that establishing collaborative relationships even in this confined environment is a skill rather than an issue of personality or 'human nature'. She undertook a forcefield analysis (*see* Appendix 2) with the staff to identify ways of reducing the tension between them and set about improving involvement and communication by developing the five projects, each of which was clearly focused on the aim of service improvement.

Case 2

THE ANOREXIA UNIT provides a nurse-led outpatient service for people with anorexia nervosa. It is a new unit within a newly established mental healthcare trust. When the interviews were conducted, it was housed in cramped rooms with little space to see patients. There are four staff, including the clinical leader who is very experienced in the treatment of people with anorexia nervosa.

What was the service improvement?

The inpatient, consultant-led service had previously been the main service provision, aiming to assist patients recover from their disorder. This facility continues with some modifications, and treatment is based on a set regime which each patient joins. The new outpatient unit has extended the range of services for people suffering from anorexia nervosa. Different kinds of treatment are offered all in one place, so that patients can have access to counselling, discuss their diets and be given practical help (e.g., with shopping) by one nurse with whom they can establish an ongoing relationship. This new approach to the service is much valued by patients and is more cost-effective for those who do not require inpatient treatment.

What was the change?

The outpatient service provided by the new unit is nurse-led, with the doctor being involved in the preliminary assessment of the patient to establish diagnosis and possible suitability for this type of treatment. The treatment goals are more varied than for the inpatient unit; the patient herself/himself decides on the outcome she or he wants, which may include finding a way of living more easily with the disorder (although there is a careful and subtle balance between patient choice and professional responsibility for ensuring that a patient is in a fit state to exercise that choice). This expanded service and the nurse-led unit have greatly extended the decision-making powers of the nurses. It has also involved some significant changes in the beliefs underlying the work concerning patient choice, and has inevitably led to system changes both in organising referral, assessment and treatment and in deciding what constitutes success.

What were the triggers for change?

The change was initiated by the clinical leader, using her knowledge of what patients want and her experience of managing the disorder. The timing of it was triggered by the opportunity provided by the King's Fund to set up an NDU.

How was the change introduced?

There was enormous difficulty in setting up this NDU to establish the new service. 'All of the gardening books say that preparing the ground is the most important and arduous part of the task,' writes the clinical leader in the unit's first Annual Report, adding that the ground had borne 'an uncanny resemblance to quicksand for much of the time'. Management uncertainties arising from the establishment of the mental health trust were combined with the retirement of the consultant leading the anorexia service, who had an international reputation.

The NDU has had to vie with other priorities on the management agenda in setting up the new trust. In fact, it was omitted from the original trust application document and the team had to seek assistance from the King's Fund to hold the trust to its original staffing commitment for the unit. While a steering group of key stakeholders led the project, the lack of a clear base for the new work has been symbolised by continuing difficulties in reaching agreement on suitable permanent accommodation for the unit.

Staff development, including induction and team-building in this small specialised team which provides an intensive service in overcrowded conditions, has constituted an important part of the change.

Case 3

AT THE TIME OF THE INTERVIEWS, the Health Visitor Unit, in which there were 13 health visitors, worked within a Community Health trust in an area of high deprivation on a large pre-war council estate.

What was the service improvement?

The focus of the team was on poverty and its impact on health and health improvements. The team aimed to move beyond an individual approach to health, where the emphasis was on child health surveillance, to working also with groups in the community to identify and act upon local health priorities. So the factors contributing to health were increasingly to become defined by the people who were themselves affected, rather than by professionals, and resources could be targetted to areas and groups in greatest need, rather than aiming for a universal service. This move to a public health focus was the change particularly discussed with the team ('Shifting conventional roles into uncharted waters', Annual Report 1994).

What was the change?

The staff developed a range of community-based activities to highlight public health issues and research these more fully for specific communities. They set up what were effectively a series of pilot projects to work on the links between poverty and health within specific groups, especially women. The unit was reorganised to create a full-time public health post from within the existing budget, to express the commitment to resourcing their new approach to health visiting.

What were the triggers for change?

The NDU was set up as a means of attracting staff to an area of work with a history of chronic staff shortages, in the context of a review of what health visiting could achieve. It was proposed that health visitors should have three functions – family health promotion, high intervention work and public health – and that this unit should try out new strategies in these three areas. This approach was fully supported by senior managers and the unit's health visitor team.

How was the change introduced?

The team were involved in intensive workshops to review their practice. To enable one health visitor to concentrate on public health aspects, her caseload was shared out among the other staff. Early activities were chosen which had an immediate high local profile (such as the accident prevention project stemming from research by the District Health Authority) and which contributed to a longer-term review (such as the community profile, based on information gathered area by area on levels of poverty and on the link between poverty and people's health). As the service development proceeded, a large number of projects were begun, some focusing on women's health or on accident prevention, others contributing to provision for children, campaigning to increase local resources or dealing with smoking and solvent abuse. All activities were based on teamwork between the health visitors and collaboration with agencies working in the area.

Case 4

THE NEIGHBOURHOOD HEALTHCARE UNIT is based in a large local healthcare trust which has developed a wide range of project work with the local communities in what is an extremely deprived inner city area. The case study focuses on one of these projects, the nutrition workshop. This workshop takes place in the crèche/waiting room at the health centre. Once a week a group of Bangladeshi women and health workers meet to discuss and write down Bangladeshi recipes, talk about healthy food and weaning babies, and try out art/design activities that relate to nutrition (such as making shapes from rice flour cakes to use as a basis for a series of embroideries; these will become part of a national multi-cultural arts initiative and exhibition).

What was the service improvement?

There is still an alarming degree of malnourishment among young Bangladeshi children in this country and health visitors recognised that their advice had not so far enabled Bangladeshi mothers to wean their children satisfactorily. The project aimed to help health workers develop ways of working that would provide the healthcare the Bangladeshi community needs but would not get without changes in health practice.

What was the change?

The change concerns the location of expertise and the move towards a partnership model based on sharing knowledge. It involves professionals saying: 'We don't know'. The nurse manager says it meant recognising that 'the base of professional knowledge is incomplete, misinformed, may be based on inaccurate information.' The workshop acts as a focus group to gain information on beliefs and practices about weaning and to document, *with* Bangladeshi women, food preparation practices and decisions about food 'to gain a more composite picture of nutrition'. One member of the unit said: 'We are teaching them about our food as well, learning both ways.' But the change also involves passing this information back to the community and finding out how the community wants it used. The staff form empathetic bonds with the Bangladeshi women. 'They are a witness even if they can't change things.' One of the Bangladeshi women attending the workshop related that after three of her children had died she had a fourth, who had difficulty feeding; the health visitor did not give specific advice, but 'would sit for hours, watch me feed and cook; she gave me encouragement whatever I did. '

What were the triggers for change?
There were a number of local triggers. Principally, the staff were building on previous work in the Health Centre which had focused on finding effective ways to 'consult the user'. Consultation meetings were not found to be the best way to consult Bangladeshi women whose public activities are limited both by their own community expectations and by the risk of racist violence. In addition, asking individuals to 'represent' their community can become tokenistic; they may feel 'privileged' at being asked and there is the risk that they will say what they think the 'authorities' want to hear. The centre had already used videotaping methods to enable local people to contribute to the identification of health needs to inform planning and purchasing. To develop further, the unit collaborated with another nutrition project launched by a local Asian women's centre and also established links with a new community arts project.

How was the change introduced?
The work was started by taking advantage of a small new funding opportunity and getting the support of middle-management in the use of premises for workshops. The project has involved an unorthodox mixture of activities carried out in an integrated way within the workshops. It has also explicitly embraced the

model of 'grounded practice', a new research practice based on partnership rather than a divide between the people who are seen as the objects of research and those carrying out the research on them. The method used in the workshops was to share activities and learning between all the people involved. This required careful attention to staff development to facilitate the group work. The team have also been working to feed what they have learned about health needs into the local purchasers' plans, to influence the new outcome-based thinking on funding healthcare in their area.

Case 5

THE ORTHOPAEDIC TRAUMA UNIT consists of two wards in a city centre teaching hospital, catering mainly for elderly patients, many of whom have a range of other chronic illnesses and conditions. The ward teams work closely with the A&E department and with community nurses and social workers on such issues as discharge (which is becoming more complex given the trends of increasing age and frailty in the elderly) and care in the community. The imminent amalgamation with an orthopaedic trauma ward at another (general) hospital added a sense of disruption and uncertainty for staff and had an impact on the progress of their service improvement project.

What was the service improvement?

The aim was to move from the existing primary nursing system to care management, using the *case management* [23] approach which originated in the USA. This involves one nurse co-ordinating all the care for a patient, following him or her through all departments and across disciplines as the 'case manager', whether or not this nurse provides direct hands-on care. It was hoped that this approach would reduce the continuity problems of managing patient care, as well as reducing lengthy stays in hospital and the resulting discharge and rehabilitation problems. The approach was seen by various key people as: improving the quality of care, reducing time spent in hospital, enabling patients to achieve rehabilitation goals more quickly, attracting fewer complaints and providing more satisfaction.

What was the change?

The unit's approach to case management involved working out a standard description of the treatment for one particular type of case over a specific timescale. This is known as a 'care-map'. Instead of patient notes, a care-map is drawn up which lists the requirements from the patient's point of view, such as information needs, pain management and wound dressing. It also sets out potential problems and standard times within which certain outcomes are normally achieved. Patients are cared for using the care-map as a guideline, and the case manager departs from it only if patients make far better or worse progress than envisaged. These patients are monitored and reasons for variations noted, in order to improve future care.

What were the triggers for change?

The change was a nurse-led initiative to extend the professional model of nursing practice and accountability which had been developed through task, then team and then primary nursing. The care-maps incorporate improvements to care, not just the mapping of the status quo, and therefore aiming to achieve higher quality of care was also important. The nurse manager saw a link between the Department of Health's Strategy for Nursing proposals, future scenarios of the Supported Early Discharge system and 'inreach' to hospitals from the community care system. The project fitted in with the hospital's interest in research and its application for NDU status and with the clinical leader's desire to develop visibly leading-edge practice. Although the care-map approach had originally been developed in the USA for cost control and as a tool for outcome-based measurement, these issues were not a trigger for change here.

How was the change introduced?

To ensure a thorough research and practice approach, a researcher was appointed to work with the clinical leader and unit staff. The first phase required undertaking a literature review on the concept of case management and US experiences with it, involving all the staff in a series of reading groups. This phase led staff to identify the need for care-maps. The unit started with one particular type of case and developed two care-maps for this, a standard one and one for 'fast-track' patients (those who were able to make a quicker recovery in their own homes). Making contact with a leading US researcher and seeking training and advice helped staff to 'sort out our care-maps, especially the length of stay'. Care-maps were developed with staff of all grades who were identified as being 'key motivated people'. They consulted other departments on the drafts and negotiated an agreed version. Medical staff were not very visibly involved in this process. During the pilot stage, both new and old systems ran in parallel, causing some stress. Conflicts between research staff and practitioners occurred over timing of implementation and over baseline data collection which nurses saw as delaying the start of the project. 'We've been waiting [for case management] for a year ... it seemed we'd never use it [work on care-maps] all.' When visited, the staff were in the very early stages of using care-maps but even at that stage one nurse said: ' I like it ... we've followed [the case] through ... it cuts the documentation.' The change happened at a time when there were many more demands than usual on staff, resulting in slow progress and inadequate management focus on the change.

Case 6

THE DISTRICT NURSING UNIT is based on the district nursing staff and their work with a community hospital trust and GP practices in an urban/rural setting. The hospital operates two general GP wards and the unit has been actively linking these and the elderly care ward to the district nursing team. The district nursing service had also been innovative in its approach to care, training and carrying out massage techniques and other complementary therapies.

What was the service improvement?

The unit set up a primary nursing system where the district nurses oversee care for their patients when they come into the hospital, although they do not carry out hands-on care as a primary nurse on the ward would do (primary nursing has been in place on wards since 1992) and as they themselves do when the patients are in their own homes. The benefits to patients and relatives include continuity of care (especially vital for pre-terminal patients) and of information. One of the district nurses said: 'Patients like the continuity of care ... can deal with complaints quickly too. They see the close relationship of nurses and see they are not abandoned by us.' Generally, the district nurses feel that there has been more and better communication and that their role as the person in charge of the care is accepted. (In parallel, they are also developing other aspects of their role, such as nursing beds, nurse prescribing and self-medication.)

What was the change?

Documentation for the district nurses as primary nurses has been developed and is in place, and one patient has gone through the new system. District nurses feel that this change recognises their previous ad hoc practice and that ward nurses have responded well to the change, resulting in better communication between the two groups. They also appreciate the changed GP role; GPs take responsibility for the drugsheet which goes with the patient to the hospital, making transfer easier, and they also consult the district nurse about discharge.

What were the triggers for change?

The desire to build up the district nurse role was a vital part of the application for NDU status and came from management (the community services manager is an ex-district nurse), from doctors (one of whom said it was 'local culture to support community hospital beds – highly valued as good for doctors and patients') and from district nurses (who are very open to new ideas, are aware of their strengths and regard themselves as 'ideally situated' for multi-disciplinary work). The basic idea stemmed specifically from one nurse informally helping a patient who was afraid of returning to hospital. The person's husband said he might be able to persuade her to go to hospital if the district nurse could still look after her. This was arranged by the district nurse and worked so well it triggered the idea of formalising the process. This nurse became the unit clinical leader. The change also benefited from the fact that key players among the district nurses were well known and respected in the hospital and by GPs, with a record of development of care and of challenging useless rules and practices. Although the community services manager wished to promote cost efficiency, the change was built on a community model of care, not on cost measures. The drawing of district nurses into the work undertaken in the wards was in tune with the shift to care in the community and linked with the trust's business plan for community-based services. The supportive community services manager was therefore able to play a key role and worked to help manage resistance among ward staff. The change will be extended to other areas since it fits the trust's objectives, and thus will not fade away if key people leave.

How was the change introduced?

The unit became an NDU at the same time as the original move to primary nursing on the wards. It was 'all too quick,' commented the nurse manager, a sentiment echoed by nurses in the ward who said it was 'too much at once'. The subsequent extension of primary nursing was not seen by district nurses as a big change: 'We visited our patients anyway'. The GPs said that the change simply 'formalised an understanding which pre-existed'. People agreed to change perhaps without knowing what was involved; ward staff and GPs were unsure of benefits at the start. The clinical leader and the community services manager attended the joint sub-committee meeting of GPs and organised a roadshow for all practices, asking for views. Other activities included a meeting with staff, development sessions and work shadowing from ward to district and vice versa, also involving night staff. The community services manager 'straddled the fence' (between hospital and community services, as she managed both). Initially, ward staff 'felt threatened' and did not like the new documentation. However, they now see that it works, with one patient having gone through the system. A monthly working party meeting on the change is still held with staff from the ward, the district and the elderly care unit. While all this is positive, some ward nurses have expressed cynicism about the change and have felt overwhelmed by the need daily to operate with insufficient resources. District nurses feel the study days (led by a known and trusted facilitator) helped ward and night staff overcome fears and accept the bringing of two cultures together into one team.

Case 7

THE DAY WARD UNIT operates within a general hospital from cramped but peaceful rooms on the top floor. Most of the patients come in for a series of oncology treatments and for endoscopies. There is an increasing speed of change in the unit's work, with pressure for more treatments, especially chemotherapies. These are now more intensive and complex, involving more procedures and patient visits and requiring more advice and post-care work (on side effects, for example). The ward has a regulated work flow with a regular patient group but there is also a constant stream of new patients who are very anxious and need a lot of time and support.

What was the service improvement?

The previous situation for these treatments involved an ad hoc arrangement whereby patients came into the outpatient department and could spend the whole day waiting to see a junior doctor who would perform the required procedure. They received no continuity of care and experienced considerable stress. In addition, the junior doctors were often not experienced in the treatments. The establishment of the day ward was intended to improve this situation, which the nurses felt was not a service at all, by providing dedicated service provision led by nursing staff who would carry out the treatments and procedures. The resulting day ward is seen by the clinical leader as a 'stimulating' place to work in and as 'nurse-led with consultant support – we are lucky with our consultants here'. There is a marked culture of excellent care, with nothing, including the demands of consultants, being allowed to stand in the way of the standards the unit sets for interaction with and care for the patients. This initiative is seen as a great success and has attracted use by 12 consultants for an increasing range of day treatments and diagnostic procedures.

What was the change?

The changes discussed with the unit were the original change to a nurse-led day ward and related subsequent developments, mainly extensions of the number and types of treatments offered and the introduction of a ward-specific computer system. This database provides a time-based record of patient care as well as rapid access to data, including information from other departments such as the 'path lab'. The new day ward involves nursing staff in scheduling, organising and carrying out a range of treatments and procedures for the patients, in liaison with the relevant consultants. They also advise patients on their treatments, especially regarding side effects. They have rapidly expanded from primarily undertaking endoscopy work to offering services in haematology and for patients with breast or bowel cancer.

What were the triggers for change?

Seven years ago nurses initiated the change to have treatments nurse-administered to improve services to patients and reduce the reliance on inexperienced junior doctors. Currently, the increasing workload caused by expanding treatment demands ('the workload is escalating – it goes in bursts') is pushing more change. The nurses took on work with lymphodema patients in 1994 and, prior to that, treatments for patients with bowel and ovarian cancer. The patterns of work seem to be changing too, with treatments bunching together more for a patient as a result of clinical developments. This is affecting workload and patterns of working.

How was the change introduced?

For the change to the nurse-led service, nurses organised their own education and training and developed new practices such as a patient appointment system and a support network or 'friendship group', linking old and new patients. Now they see themselves as experts in the field. The range of procedures takes time to learn, with particularly high demands at first. In addition, it is hard to get busy staff to take time to teach the procedures as they are under pressure and, as one ward nurse commented, 'the consultants want it perfect.' Money, 'even small amounts', was a key element in getting change to happen. The funding from the King's Fund enabled them to acquire the computer. This aspect of the change was developed in collaboration with hospital information technology staff, and acted as a kind of pilot project for both groups. Although it has been through 80 amendments, the computer system seems 'owned' by the unit compared with other wards which will receive a system they have not helped to develop. The computer gives them 'hard data' with which to argue the case for resources; it analyses treatment volumes rather than patient numbers, which is a more accurate reflection of activity and helps to calculate staff hours. However, staff have to organise the time themselves to learn to use it. With regard to the shift to scheduling work for themselves, the clinical leader said: 'We are well organised but also have to be flexible.' They have reached the unusual situation of being in control of bed allocation to ensure the efficient use of beds, rather than working around set days for particular consultants, as at the outset.

Case 8

THE MATERNITY UNIT is based in a large new general hospital. It was established as a new unit when the hospital opened in 1992.

What was the service improvement?

The service has shifted from a fairly traditional consultant-led, high-intervention approach to maternity services, with one service for all women, to a differentiated service. The NDU offers mid-wife-led services to 'low-risk' women in a caring, 'low-tech' and deliberately calm environment. Each woman sees the consultant only once, at 16 weeks (although the value of even this session is currently under review). Women identified as high risk are referred to a different hospital, where the service is oriented to more complex cases and is still consultant-led. The unit is also moving towards integrating the hospital and community midwife teams to develop further the continuity of care and offer the best range of choices to women in the district.

What was the change?

The unit went through a major and radical change on moving to the new site, which coincided with the shift to a midwife-led service and to sending higher-risk women to another unit. The biggest change was in the level of responsibility for the senior midwives, who took on a role on a par with that of consultants in relation to the low-risk women. Within specific criteria (and the consultants' continuing overall clinical responsibility for the women in the unit and their diagnosis as 'low risk' or not), the midwives decide on drugs, mode of birth and subsequent care with the women, as well as carrying out suturing. Continually exploring and monitoring this shift of responsibility has been key to the change being implemented.

What were the triggers for change?

The major trigger was a threat to close down the maternity unit in order to rationalise the service to the other major hospital in the district. The resulting public campaign supported by mothers, GPs and the National Childbirth Trust, as well as by the midwives, had a great impact on decisions. It also benefited from the focus on the NHS in the impending general election. The campaign was won by the proposal to offer a different service, one solely for low-risk women. The other important component was the national maternity services review, 'Changing Childbirth', which supported the shift to increasing women's choices and strengthening the role of midwives.

How was the change introduced?

The change to the midwife-led unit was a major and radical one, happening effectively overnight with the unit's move to the new hospital premises in early 1992. 'On reflection, we should have closed the ward,' commented the clinical leader. This move had followed not only the campaigning described above but also intensive work with all the women in the 6 weeks leading up to the move. It involved a great deal of work after the move, requiring long hours and strong commitment by staff to make the new system work. Many after-hours meetings were held and the midwives had to feel their way towards operating norms in terms of their new responsibilities. They checked a great deal with registrars to start with and felt they were under observation for failure. The new autonomy was frightening at the start and, to some extent, these stresses continue. One midwife commented: 'I still feel we are being watched. We can so easily be labelled an unsafe unit.' Following the massive momentum of the first nine months or so, the staff experienced a 'dip' and talked of feeling 'tired', 'disgruntled' and 'floundering'. The nurse manager deliberately slowed the pace of change, 'let things drift for a bit' and then refocused the staff through projects such as business planning and G grade sisters meetings. The changes that are continuing (such as integrating the teams) are being tackled in a more 'evolutionary' way. A consultant said: 'Each step must be acceptable to GPs.' Managing change for this unit has always been strongly linked to the views of all the interest groups, and remains an important aspect. Increasingly, this means working through and with the purchaser of maternity services, using the unit's expertise and information about user needs to influence the shape and size of the future services.

Appendix 2
Analytical frameworks

The three analytical frameworks mentioned in the text are outlined here. These frameworks can be useful in analysing organisational contexts and programmes for action. They are:

- power net analysis
- forcefield analysis
- SWOT analysis.

Power net analysis [24]

A crucial aspect of getting things done, through meetings or in other ways, is understanding organisational politics and power. Who will help and who will hinder you, and why? What will influence people to support you and your aims?

The exercise of power involves person A influencing person B to do what A wants. If you ask: 'Why will B do what A wants?', the answer will give a measure of the power of A. While A can be seen to have sources of power to influence B, B usually also has some power; politics is seldom a one-way system, and it can also shift radically over time as things change.

Type and source of power

These are complex and often overlapping to a large degree. They are also subject to issues of *prior inequality* between people, especially in relation to groups who are usually excluded. People at work will therefore have power according to their attributes of gender, 'race', physical ability/ disability, class, education, age and sexuality. Their power will also be determined by the following factors:

- *Formal authority* – the right to make decisions conferred on you by higher management and/or your allocated role in the organisation. It depends on people's acceptance of your right to decide, and is seldom sufficient on its own, but is usually found in conjunction with one or more of the other types or sources of power.

- *Expertise* – specialist knowledge and skills, usually acquired through professional training outside the organisation. The more exclusive your expertise and the more useful it is seen to be in the organisation, the more power it confers.

- *Resources* – control of physical, financial or information resources. People in relatively low positions in the hierarchy can have considerable resource power. Most power goes to those who control the most valued resources, particularly money and information. Information is one of the most important political resources and requires attention to informal as well as formal channels in order to manage its power.

- *Personal attributes* – the ability to persuade and to build good relationships. This ability depends on personal flair as well as on the skills gained through experience, training and conscious practice.

- *Gatekeeping* – control of access to people, information, resources and decision-makers. This is a barrier or stopping power and can be especially negative and destructive.

You can illustrate your own power situation by drawing a power net, with you in the middle and other key people (those who have an important effect on you and your work) around you (*see* Figure 3). They may be higher or lower than you in the hierarchy and inside or outside the organisation. In the diagram, label each link with the type and source of power between you and these key people, and between them and you. Remember that power often flows both ways.

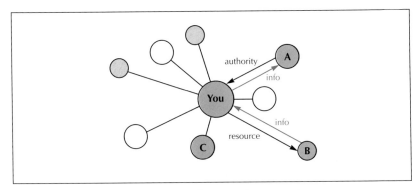

Fig. 3: *Developing a 'power net'*

Forcefield analysis [25]

This is a simple but widely used framework to help plan changes in a way that makes explicit what you are probably thinking about in any case. It is based on Kurt Lewin's idea. That no situation is entirely immovable and that the forces which define a situation are fluid and dynamic, rather than fixed, and can be influenced. The analysis involves four stages:

Stage 1   Identify the change that you want to bring about. Write down this specific change. If it is a complex all-encompassing change, it can be helpful to break it down into more specific changes.

Stage 2   Think about the existing forces that are helping this change to happen, and those that are preventing or inhibiting it. These forces may be societal factors, specific groups or individual people. Draw a diagram to illustrate these forces (*see* Figure 4).

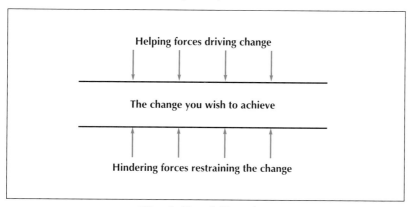

Fig. 4: Forcefield analysis

Stage 3   This stage is about what you can do. Start with the forces which are preventing or inhibiting the change. Take each one and decide whether there is anything you can do to reduce the strength of this force, and if so, what. Write this on the diagram. Then look at the helping forces, and decide what you can do to enhance them, if anything? Write these actions on the diagram.

Stage 4   Assess the whole diagram and work out which actions you think are the most feasible and most useful. From these, write an action plan, with a timescale attached.

SWOT analysis

'SWOT' stands for 'Strengths, Weaknesses, Opportunities and Threats'. The SWOT technique, developed at Harvard Business School and often used in a marketing context, enables an environmental analysis to be made of an organisation. Such an analysis should be a key component of the strategic or business plan in order to prevent a static and narrow view of the organisation's strategy.

Strengths and weaknesses are related to the *internal* environment of an organisation. Opportunities and threats are related to its *external* environment (often referred to as the market analysis). The technique requires you to list issues as specifically as you can under each heading, taking time to *compile each list separately,* so as not to muddle issues together. Some items may appear in two lists (e.g., something may be both a threat and a potential opportunity).

It is important to specify *how* the items are strengths, threats, opportunities or threats. For example, putting purchasers as a threat is not specific enough to be useful. What is it that makes them a threat? Is it their strong views on priorities or their lack of understanding of the service you are offering?

Figure 5 illustrates SWOT analysis and its elements. Use of this diagram will help to ensure that you have considered all the key environmental factors in your SWOT analysis.

SWOT analysis is also a tool to use with other stakeholders such as staff and users. It is important to try to obtain a broad view, especially of strengths and weaknesses, rather than rely on your own management view. Be open to all the information available; this will help in carrying out a special survey if this kind of critical self analysis is new to your organisation or unit.

Once you have as full an analysis as possible, you will be ready to review the results of the analysis and begin to identify the strategic issues which need to be addressed in your action plan. The idea is to consider all the ideas together and to pinpoint the key issues which emerge overall. These should then become the major strategic concerns of the plan. You may also identify elements in the SWOT analysis

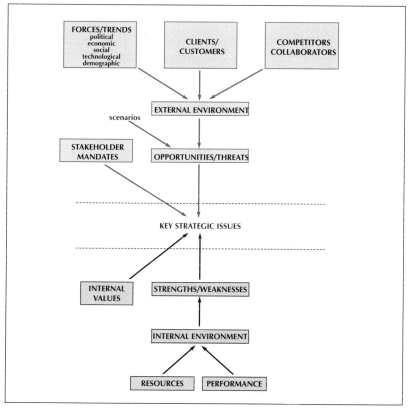

Source: Adapted from Bryson & Roering. Applying Private Sector Planning in the Public Sector. 1987; *APA Journal*, Winter.

Fig. 5: 'SWOT' *analysis*

which you feel you cannot influence. This is to be expected, so concentrate on areas where you can influence people and actions.

To focus your analysis, ask the following questions:

• what are the strategic issues we must address?
• what must we do well to achieve the change we want?
• what strengths should we build on and/or exploit?
• what weaknesses must we tackle?
• what opportunities should we develop?
• what threats must we counteract or minimise?

And then agree on *the key strategic goals you should set to tackle your service improvement.*

Chapter 1

Whether the approach to introducing change is incremental or radical, the case studies show that *from the outset the whole process needs to be visualised within a broad strategic context, with clear goals.* What is required is a strategy that takes into account not only the systems but also the staff, the structures and the management style (*see* Figure 1).

Within this overall approach to change, getting the speed of the actual change right for the people involved is crucial to prevent them being overwhelmed with too rapid a change or bored with a process that never seems to end.

What has emerged from the case studies is that the change strategist[4] (in these cases, usually the ward sister or clinical leader) needs to *plan for the change and try to envisage how it will affect the people involved.* The strategist also needs to communicate fully at all stages with everyone involved, paying particular attention to people still on the edge of the change so that they know what to expect and when. These skills were developed through a learning process over time, through discussions and analysis with colleagues, facilitated by the King's Fund project officers.

The comments made by the clinical leader of the Maternity Unit on strategic planning indicate that the effort required to make changes had not been predicted: 'That's something to be learned: trying to have a more strategic approach as a manager... On reflection, we should have closed the ward... It was very busy, senior midwives had to learn to cope with that responsibility. This provided momentum for the next few months. Staff were very committed, they had evening meetings outside duty hours and stayed late. This lasted 9 to 12 months. Then staff became disgruntled. They were tired and they did not want to change any more. People started floundering.'

Another clinical leader acknowledged the lack of strategic planning thus: 'Setting up the NDU was seen as a way to recruit staff to a hard-to-recruit area ... [there was] no framework of stages we need to go through ... that [process of] learning has been invaluable for me.'

The initial analysis of the case studies highlighted the key issues in introducing changes aimed at service improvement:

- successful change requires *systematic attention to all the aspects* of the change and recognition of their interconnectedness; the 'Seven S' model may be useful as a checklist for what needs to considered about aspects of the change being planned
- drawing up an *explicit strategic plan* at the outset helps a great deal, particularly in terms of deciding whether the radical or incremental approach is best and identifying the strengths and weaknesses of each approach
- consideration needs to be given to *the speed of the change and its impact* on all the people involved, especially the recipients of change[5] who are usually the people who will need to carry out the new activities
- communication about the change needs to *spell out the process of the change as well as the content of the change* (i.e., its clinical or practice content).

The case studies also underlined the importance of outside factors in managing change. These are considered in more depth in Chapter 2.

Chapter 2

Successful innovators had undertaken an explicit analysis of their key stakeholders and identified the stakeholders' areas of interest and the criteria upon which they would judge the unit. These innovators were also aware of the gender and 'race'[8] issues involved and how they would affect (though not govern) stakeholders' interests and powers. This enabled them to practise what might be called 'stakeholder management': with a clear picture of the differing interests and powers involved, they worked with the stakeholders to help them contribute to and support the service improvement. Where innovators had *not* 'managed' key stakeholders, problems emerged.

This chapter looked at ways of managing change that helped nurse managers achieve their aims, and raised some of the difficulties which hindered them; these are discussed further in Chapter 3.

In their study on organisational change, Moss Kanter, Stein and Jick[9] suggest that in the change process there are three main groups of participants:

- change strategists, who look at the connection between the organisation and its environment
- change implementers, who are responsible for the internal organisational implications of introducing changes
- change recipients, who are affected by the change and react to it.

The key issue here is that these roles need not be held by separate individuals, although there may be a difference in perspective. Nurses often feel that they are implementers and recipients, rarely strategists. However, those introducing change in the units studied have clearly acted as change strategists as well as implementers in that they recognised that successful service improvement involves the following steps:

1 Identify the key people whose support for the change is needed (stakeholders) and assess their interest in the improvement
2 Treat stakeholders as an 'invisible team' who are vital to the success of the project and therefore need to be kept informed and involved
3 Plan and organise ways of gathering data from and/or with stakeholders, taking account of gender and 'race' issues
4 Analyse and market the strengths of the project, especially nurses' skills and expert knowledge (particularly knowledge of service users and their needs) and identify any weaknesses in order to counteract them
5 Be pro-active in using external factors where they are relevant to the change by looking for opportunities and threats in the wider environment, outside the unit
6 Keep a firm focus on the overall aims of the change by working to an explicit strategic plan
7 Pursue the plan actively, ensuring that the key stakeholders, including purchasers and senior managers, understand the plan and are kept informed of its progress through maintaining dialogue with them.

All these elements appear in general 'recipes' for managing change, but the case studies showed that they are both necessary and yet can be difficult to achieve at operational level for nurse managers. The key principles so far identified from the case studies all illustrate *the importance of adopting a strategic approach to achieving service improvement,* no matter how small the change may appear to be.

Chapter 3

The issues raised in this chapter are primarily for individual nurse managers to consider and analyse in order to set development goals for themselves or in consultation with their supervisors. But the wider issues raised about the links between nursing, management, gender, 'race' and other organisational issues also need to be considered by those in the profession who are developing the nurse role overall, as well as the training and education this requires. They also pose a clear challenge to trust management in developing organisational structures and culture.

The conclusion from the case studies is that, for successful change in service provision, nurses need to recognise and develop their management role. This requires:

- giving constant consideration to the *organisational aspects* of the change, as well as the clinical elements which are naturally their first focus
- focusing on *managing outwards* as well as inside their unit
- identifying their strengths and *publishing the achievements* of their work in their own institution (and more widely, if possible)
- bringing into their management practice the *hidden or absent dimensions* relating to gender, 'race', disability and sexuality when developing service improvements.

Chapter 4

Managing paradoxes is an inescapable part of public sector management. The cases demonstrated a number of ways of embedding change that help to chart a course through these paradoxes. The constancy of change, especially in the external environment, also requires a nurse manager to take chances, create opportunities and use resources fully.

When planning or considering a service improvement, it is important at the outset to assess which approaches would be most likely to embed the change. The main issues to consider are:

- the way in which the *type of service improvement* may itself suggest a procedural or cultural approach
- the need to build on this and consider *what gaps* might be left to be filled

- the value of recognising and *working with strengths in personal management style* (e.g., in organising groups of stakeholders) and at the same time recognising areas needing more attention (e.g., in applying a procedural approach to embedding change, such as gaining formal acknowledgement from trust managers)
- working with stakeholders to *develop new ways*, not mentioned in this study, to embed changes
- the importance of a *partnership* relationship with the purchaser.

It is becoming increasingly important to ask, throughout the change process: *How else* could we do this? Seeking answers to this question stimulates creativity and positive response to opportunities which are vital elements of a strategic management repertoire.

Chapter 5

The purpose of this chapter is to identify ways in which nurse managers can apply a strategic approach to service improvement. Drawing on observations in the units studied, the discussion looks at successful approaches to providing a better experience for patients or clients and how these approaches differed from 'coping management'. It also examines some of the assumptions underlying the organisation of healthcare work which may make strategic approaches to management difficult for nurses.

Some of these assumptions, such as the division of labour between nurses and doctors, were being challenged in productive ways in the units visited, but others, such as 'male' and 'female' patterns of work, went unmentioned and unchallenged. When assumptions remain unexamined, they can contribute to what is termed the 'organisational neglect' of nursing and make it more difficult for nurse managers to change the structures of service delivery. This chapter offers specific suggestions on how to uncover and challenge such assumptions.

Writers in many fields of management have tried to define the term 'strategic', but there is little agreement except that it is a multi-faceted rather than single concept. Having a strategic focus means both having a particular attitude, a set of tools and techniques, and a process for managing. The suggestions for strategic action given here embrace all these and offer learning from the case studies as a starting point for further development and learning in readers' own organisations.

Notes

1   The term 'nurse manager' is used as well as 'clinical leader' as this study was concerned with the *management* role of nurses, in addition to other roles some of them carried out. In some cases, clinical leaders were also line managers; in other cases, the roles were split. This proved to be an important distinction.

2   Pascale R. *Managing on the edge: How successful companies use conflict to stay ahead.* Harmondsworth, Middlesex: Penguin, 1990. Page 40.

3   Quinn JB. Managing strategies incrementally. *Omega: International Journal of Management Science* 1982

4   Moss Kanter R, Stein B, Jick T. *The challenge of organisational change: How companies experience it and leaders guide it.* New York: Free Press, 1992. Pages 14-17.

5   *See* 4.

6   *See* discussion on 'coping management' in Chapter 5.

7   Pettigrew A, Ferlie E, McKee L. *Shaping strategic change.* London: Sage, 1992.

8   The term 'race' is used in inverted commas throughout in order to indicate the complexity of the construction of racial identity.

9   *See* 4.

10 Hastings C, Bixby P, Chaudhry-Lawton R. *Superteams: A blueprint for organisational success.* Fontana/Collins, 1986. Page 43.

11 Robinson K, Vaughan B. *Knowledge for nursing practice.* Oxford: Butterworth–Heinemann, 1992. Chapter 1.

12 Illich I. Vernacular values. In Kumar S, Blond, Briggs (eds.) *Schumacher Lectures* 1980.

13 Moss Kanter R. *Men and women of the corporation.* Unwin, 1977.

14 'The Tale of O.' 1980. A videotape produced by Goodmeasure Inc., Cambridge, MA, USA.

15 Goodman and Dean. Creating long-term organisational change. In Goodman (ed.) *Change in Organisations.* Jossey Bass, 1982. Page 268.

16 Mintzberg H. Crafting strategy. *Harvard Business Review* July–August 1987.

17 *See* 2.

18 Davies C. Gender, history and management style in nursing: Towards a theoretical synthesis. In Savage M, Witz A. (eds.) *Gender and bureaucracy.* Oxford: Blackwell, Page 238.

19 *See* 18. Page 245.

20 Weil S. *Enhancing clinical effectiveness through continuous professional development and clinical audit.* NHS Clinical Outcomes Group, 1994 (Unpublished).

21 Harlow E, Hearn J, Parkin W. Gendered noise and the silence and din of domination. In Itzin C. and Newman J. (eds.) *Gender, culture and organisational change.* London: Routledge, 1995

22 *See* 7. Page 8.

23 Petryshen P, Petryshen P. The case management model: An innovative approach to the delivery of patient care. *Journal of Advanced Nursing* 1992; 17:1168–94.

24 Adapted from the training work of Reena Bhownani and the discussion in Handy C. *Understanding organisations.* Harmondsworth, Middlesex: Penguin Education, 1976. Pages 118-29 and 436-9.

25 Lewin K. Frontiers in group dynamics: concept, method and reality in social sciences: social equilibria and social change. *Human Relations.* 1947; 1(1): 5-41.